Toxoplasmosis

NATO ASI Series

Advanced Science Institutes Series

A series presenting the results of activities sponsored by the NATO Science Committee, which aims at the dissemination of advanced scientific and technological knowledge, with a view to strengthening links between scientific communities.

The Series is published by an international board of publishers in conjunction with the NATO Scientific Affairs Division

A Life Sciences	Plenum Publishing Corporation
B Physics	London and New York
C Mathematical and Physical Sciences	Kluwer Academic Publishers Dordrecht, Boston and London
D Behavioural and Social Sciences	
E Applied Sciences	
F Computer and Systems Sciences	Springer-Verlag Berlin Heidelberg New York
G Ecological Sciences	London Paris Tokyo Hong Kong
H Cell Biology	Barcelona Budapest
I Global Environmental Change	

NATO-PCO DATABASE

The electronic index to the NATO ASI Series provides full bibliographical references (with keywords and/or abstracts) to more than 30000 contributions from international scientists published in all sections of the NATO ASI Series. Access to the NATO-PCO DATABASE compiled by the NATO Publication Coordination Office is possible in two ways:

- via online FILE 128 (NATO-PCO DATABASE) hosted by ESRIN, Via Galileo Galilei, I-00044 Frascati, Italy.

- via CD-ROM "NATO Science & Technology Disk" with user-friendly retrieval software in English, French and German (© WTV GmbH and DATAWARE Technologies Inc. 1992).

The CD-ROM can be ordered through any member of the Board of Publishers or through NATO-PCO, Overijse, Belgium.

Series H: Cell Biology, Vol. 78

Toxoplasmosis

Edited by

Judith E. Smith

Department of Pure & Applied Biology
University of Leeds
Leeds LS2 9JT, U.K.

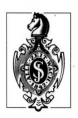

Springer-Verlag
Berlin Heidelberg New York London Paris Tokyo
Hong Kong Barcelona Budapest
Published in cooperation with NATO Scientific Affairs Division

Proceedings of the NATO Advanced Research Workshop on Toxoplasmosis, held at Fontevraud, France, June 28–July 2, 1992

QR
201
.T53
T69
1993

ISBN 3-540-57305-4 Springer-Verlag Berlin Heidelberg New York
ISBN 0-387-57305-4 Springer-Verlag New York Berlin Heidelberg

Library of Congress Cataloging-in-Publication Data.
Toxoplasmosis / edited by Judith E. Smith. p. cm. – (NATO ASI series. Series H. Cell biology; vol. 78)
"Published in cooperation with the NATO Scientific Affairs Division."
"Proceedings of the NATO Advanced Research Workshop on Toxoplasmosis, held at Fontevraud, France, June 28-July 2, 1992" – T.p. verso. Includes bibliographical references and index.
ISBN 3-540-57305-4 (alk. paper). – ISBN 0-387-57305-4 (alk. paper).
1. Toxoplasmosis–Microbiology–Congresses. 2. Toxoplasmosis–Molucular aspects–Congresses. 3. Toxoplasmosis–Immunology–Congresses. I. Smith, Judith E., 1952- . II. North Atlantic Treaty Organization. Scientific Affairs Division. III. NATO Advanced Research Workshop on Toxoplasmosis, (1992: Fontevraud-l'Abbaye, France) IV. Series. [DNLM: 1. Toxoplasmosis–congresses. WC 725 T755 1992] QR201.T53T69 1993 616.9'36–dc20 DNLM/DLC for Library of Congress 93-35674

© Springer-Verlag Berlin Heidelberg 1993
Printed in Germany

Typesetting: Camera ready by authors
31/3145 - 5 4 3 2 1 0 - Printed on acid-free paper

PREFACE

Although long known as a parasite of medical and veterinary importance, interest in *Toxoplasma gondii* has increased with its emergence as a major cause of death in immunosuppressed individuals, and with recognition of its suitability as a model system for molecular and cellular investigations of apicomplexan parasites. The NATO workshop brought together 32 scientists working in different areas of toxoplasmosis research to gain an overview of progress in the field.

Molecular studies have been carried out on genomic and extrachromosomal DNA. They reveal that *Toxoplasma* is very highly conserved, genetic mapping is underway and preliminary linkage analysis suggests recombination is rare; moreover all virulent strains share the same isoenzyme markers and are seen to be essentially clonal by RFLP analysis [Boothroyd, Darde, Wilson].

Despite considerable structural homology between *Toxoplasma* and related apicomplexan parasites there is little direct overlap in gene sequence data. Good progress has been made in cloning functional genes and in elucidation of PI anchors [Cesbron-Delauw, Johnson, Mercereau-Puijalon, Striepen]. The structure of molecules on the surface and within dense granules, rhoptries and micronemes has in some cases been determined and provides clues as to the targetting and function of these proteins.

Events relating to the formation of a fusion incompetent parasitophorous vacuole have also been clarified. Host cell membrane markers are excluded from the developing PV membrane during invasion, this is followed by the synchronous, Ca^{++} dependent, release of dense granule proteins [Sibley]. One of which forms aggregates on the cytoplasmic side of the PV membrane and may be a pore forming protein responsible for enabling the free movement of small molecules [Joiner].

Study of parasite differentiation between bradyzoite and tachyzoite stages has been facilitated by *in vitro* culture. Switching between the two stages is a stochastic event involving sequential changes for individual parasites, however bradyzoite initiated cultures produce a cohort of mature cysts [Dubremetz, Smith].

Although humoral immunity is important in neutralising and destroying extracellular parasites, cellular mechanisms are now believed to be paramount.

Cell mediated protective immunity is reported following vaccination with protein and peptides of SAG1, GRA2 & ROP2 [Darcy, Herion, Kasper]. Production of gamma-IFN, of CD8$^+$ cytotoxic lymphocytes, and macrophage activation are thought to be important; as are the induction of harmful cytokine profiles, which induce tolerance & suppression [McLeod, Sher, Suzuki].

A live vaccine against congenital infection in sheep is currently in use and progress has been made in selecting suitable animal models for testing defined antigens [Bos, Alexander]. Chemotherapy, however, remains the main method of disease control, novel compounds are rare and stress should be laid on using combinations of drugs [Araujo, Chang]. Recombinant antigens and PCR based techniques are contributing to improved diagnosis [Tenter, Schoondermark-van de Ven].

ACKNOWLEDGEMENTS

We gratefully acknowledge the support of the North Atlantic Treaty Organisation (NATO) in providing funds for this meeting. We wish to thank Dr Francoise Darcy-Szekely for acting as local convenor and staff at the Hotellerie du Prieure st-Lazare, in particular M.D. Haudebaut & Mlle. M.N. Boutard, for providing excellent conference facilities, accommodation and food. In preparing the manuscripts for publication I am deeply indebted to Ms Sharon Hunter for excellent secretarial assistance and to Dr Martin Hemingway for assistance throughout.

ADVANCED SERIES WORKSHOP ON
TOXOPLASMOSIS PARTICIPANTS

ALEXANDER, James
Division of Immunology
University of Strathclyde
The Todd Centre
31 Taylor Street
Glasgow, G4 0NR
U.K.

ARAUJO, Fausto
Department of Immunology & Infectious Diseases
Research Inst Palo Alto Medical Foundation
860 Bryant Street
Palo Alto
CA 94301
U.S.A.

BLACKWELL, Jenefer M
Department of Medicine
Level 5, Addenbrookes Hospital
Hills Road, Cambridge, CB2 2QQ
U.K.

BOOTHROYD, John C
Department of Microbiology & Immunology
Stanford University
School of Medicine
Stanford CA 94305-5402

BOS, Hans J
Intervet International BV
Virology & Parasitology R & D Department
Postbox 31
5830 AA BOXMEER
The Netherlands

BOUT, Daniel
URIP
Centre INRA de TOURS
37380 Nouzilly
France

CESBRON-DELAUW, Marie-France
Centre Immunologie et de Biologie Parasitaire
INSERM U167, Institut Pasteur
1 Rue de Prof A Calmette
BP 245, 59019 Lille Cedex
France

CHANG, Hernan R
Department of Microbiology
Faculty of Medicine, National University of Singapore
Lower Kent Ridge Road
Singapore 0511

DARCY-SZEKELY, Francoise
INSERM U298
CHUD
F.49033 Angers
Cedex 01
France

DARDE, Marie-Laure
Service de Parasitologie
CHRU
2 Ave Alexis-Carrel
87042 Limoges Cedex
France

DILMEN Ugar
Turkish Health & Therapy Foundation
Medical Center Hospital
Department of Neonatology
06510 Emek, Ankara
Turkey

DUBREMETZ Jean-Francois
INSERM U42
369, rue J Guesde
BP 39 59651 Villeneuve d'Ascq Cédex
France

HERION, Pascal
Department de Immunologia
Instituto de Investigaciones Biomedicas
Universidad Nacional Autonoma de Mexico
AP 70228
Ciudad Universitaria
04510 Mexico DF
Mexico

JOHNSON, Alan
Department of Microbiology
University of Technology Sydney
Westbourne Street, Gore Hill
NSW 2007
Australia

JOINER, Keith
Department of Internal Medicine
Yale University
808 LCL, P O Box 3333
New Haven, Connecticut
06510-8056
U.S.A.

KANELLI-PAPAIOANNOU, Stamatia
Institut Pasteur Hellenique
127 vas Sofias Ave
Gr115 21 Athenes
Greece

KASPER, Lloyd
Section of Neurology
Dartmouth Medical School
2 Maynard Street
Hanover
New Hampshire 03756
U.S.A.

McLEOD, Rima
Division of Infectious Diseases
Michael Reese Medical Center
2929 S.Ellis
Chicago
Illinois 60616
U.S.A.

MERCEREAU-PUIJALON, Odile
Unite de Parasitologie Experimentale
Institut Pasteur
25 Rue de Dr Roux
75015 Paris
France

MOUGIN, Bruno
bioMerieux
22 rue St Jean-de-Dieu
69007 Lyon
France

SCHOONDERMARK-van de VEN Esther
Department of Medical Microbiology
University Hospital Nijmegen
P O Box 9101
6500 HB Nijmegen
The Netherlands

SCHWARZ, Ralph
Zentrum fur Hygiene und Medizinische Mikrobiologie
Philipps-Universitat Marburg
Robert-Koch Strasse
D-3550 Marburg
Germany

SCHWARTZMAN, Joseph
Department of Pathology
Dartmouth-Hitchcock Medical Center
Lebanon
New Hampshire 03756
U.S.A.

SEITZ, H.M.
Institute fur Medical Parasitologie
Sigmund-Freud-Strasse 25
W-5300 Bonn1
Germany

SHER, Alan
Laboratory of Parasitic Diseases
National Institute of Allergy & Infectious Diseases
NIH, Building 4, Room 126
Bethesda Maryland 20892
U.S.A.

SIBLEY, L. David
Department of Molecular Microbiology
Washington University Medical Center
Box 8230
660 South Euclid Ave
St Louis, Missouri 63110-1093
U.S.A.

SMITH, Judith
Department of Pure & Applied Biology
University of Leeds
Leeds LS2 9JT
U.K.

STREIPEN Boris
Zentrum fur Hygiene und Medizinische Mikrobiologie
Philipps-Universitat Marburg
Robert-Koch Strasse
D-3550 Marburg
Germany

SUZUKI Yasuhiro
Department of Parasitology
Jikei University School of Medicine
3-25-8 Nishi-Shinbashi
Minato-Ku
Tokyo 105, Japan

TENTER, Astrid
Institut fur Parasitologie
Tierarztliche Hockschule Hannover
Bunteweg 17
D 3000 Hannover 71
Germany

VOLPE F
Wellcome Research Laboratories
Langley Court
Beckenham
Kent BR3 3BS
U.K.

WEISS, Louis M
Department of Pathology
Albert Einstein College of Medicine
Yeshiva University
Jack & Pearl Resnick Campus
1300 Morris Park Avenue
Bronx New York 10461
U.S.A.

WILSON, Iain
NIMR
The Ridgeway
Mill Hill
London, NW7 1AA
U.K.

CONTENTS

IMMUNOLOGY

TOXOPLASMOSIS VACCINES DIAGNOSIS & CHEMOTHERAPY

MOLECULAR BIOLOGY
OF
TOXOPLASMA

ALLELIC POLYMORPHYISM IN *TOXOPLASMA GONDII* IMPLICATIONS FOR INTERSTRAIN MATING

John C. Boothroyd, Allen J. LeBlanc[*] and L. David Sibley[*]
Department of Microbiology and Immunology
Standford University School of Medicine
Stanford, CA 94305-5402 U.S.A.

Introduction

The life cycle of *Toxoplasma gondii* is complex with several alternative sub-cycles. It can, for example, pass from cat to cat through an oral-faecal route, each time going through a sexual cycle in the intestine of the cat. This sub-cycle can be considered to begin with excretion of highly stable oocysts in the faeces of an infected cat. Upon maturation, these oocysts will contain two sporocysts, each comprising four sporozoites. Transmission occurs when the mature oocysts are ingested by another cat with release of the sporozoites in the intestine.   These invade the intestinal epithelium where they divide intracellularly, ultimately differentiating into either micro- or macro-gametes. Fusion of the two gametes gives rise to the zygote which develops into the immature oocyst. The cycle is completed upon release of these oocysts into the environment. Felidae is the only genus known in which gametogenesis and oocyst production occurs.

The parasite can also reproduce via an entirely asexual sub-cycle through infection of any of a large number of land-dwelling vertebrates (i.e., mammals and birds). This cycle relies on carnivorism wherein the parasite is ingested by the carnivore in the form of tissue cysts found in various organs of the prey animal. This need not result in an inevitable spiral "up" the food chain as scavengers will readily reintroduce the parasites back into prey.

---

* present addresses:
L.D.S., Department of Molecular Microbiology, Washington University School of Medicine, St. Louis, MO63110, U.S.A.; AJL, Department of Biochemistry, University of Alabama School of Medicine, Birmingham, AL35222, U.S.A.

NATO ASI Series, Vol. H 78
Toxoplasmosis
Edited by Judith E. Smith
© Springer-Verlag Berlin Heidelberg 1993

These two sub-cycles can overlap when, for example, a grazing herbivore ingests oocysts present in the environment or when a cat preys on an infected mouse. In the latter case, the parasites contained within tissue cysts in the mouse are released and after a few rounds of multiplication can enter into the sexual cycle and gametogenesis, culminating in the production of oocysts.

The relative contribution of these different subcycles to the proliferation of Toxoplasma in nature is not known. It could be that one or other predominates or that they are all intertwined and intricately balanced. One way of examining this is to look at the frequencies of polymorphic alleles in the population. For example, at one extreme, that of almost exclusively asexual reproduction, one might find that there is strong linkage disequilibrium (i.e., loci that are not in fact linked show significant association in certain strains). On the other hand, if the sexual cycle is a frequently used part of the cycle then one might expect to find frequencies of different alleles at about that predicted if the population is in genetic equilibrium (which results from random and at least moderately frequent genetic exchange or mating).

To test this, we have previously reported on the analysis of 28 strains at each of nine loci and found that the global population of *T. gondii* shows acute linkage disequilibrium such that all virulent strains appear to be derived from a single clonal lineage. Nonvirulent strains show more diversity but even these, when analyzed as a separate group, show significant evidence of linkage disequilibrium. As already stated, linkage equilibrium requires both random and frequent mating. Hence, the results with the 28 strains could be due to either very rare or non-random mating. Here, we have analyzed three strains at each of 36 polymorphic loci to determine the extent to which these three strains share a common gene pool. The results are discussed in the context of the extent to which the virulent and nonvirulent strains are related.

Results and Discussion

Three strains were chosen for our analysis. Two of the strains, C and P are non-virulent. C was originally isolated by Elmer Pfefferkorn from a cat in Dartmouth, New Hampshire (it is sometimes referred to as CEP). P is a derivative of the ME49 strain which was first isolated from a sheep in California (it was cloned by Lloyd Kasper and is therefore sometimes referred to as PLK). These two strains have been used by us to generate a genetic map of *T. gondii* [Sibley et al., 1992] and, as they successfully mated in a cat co-infected with tissue cysts of each, they can be reasonably assumed to be members of the same species. The third train, RH, is a well-studied, virulent strain that was originally isolated from a boy in Ohio. Perhaps due to its extensive laboratory passaging, this strain is apparently not capable of entering a sexual cycle in the cat and so it is not possible to address whether it is a member of the same species as P and C strains by this simple test.

In all, 36 distinct and for the most part random, single-copy loci were examined using cDNA probes as cloned in plasmids. Each insert was radiolabelled and used in turn to probe Southern blots of genomic DNA from the three strains individually digested with each of a large number of restriction endonucleases. On average, a total of 11 enzymes were used in the analysis with each probe. In practice, this was done by reprobing a given blot, containing the digested DNA from the three strains, 5-10 times, stripping off one probe before using the next. To ensure the most accurate comparisons for each enzyme digest, the DNA from the three strains was always run in adjacent lanes.

To gain some understanding of the relationship between virulent and non-virulent strains, the data were scored in the following way. For each probe, the total number of restriction enzymes that yielded a RFLP specific to a given strain was divided by the total number of enzyme digests analyzed with that probe. The resulting decimal was multiplied by 100 to give "% strain-specific polymorphism".

The results are summarized in figure 1. The probes have been assigned to one of four groups: "non-specific" probes detect loci with little polymorphism, the other three groups represent loci that show a polymorphism specific for one or other of the three strains.

From these results, it is clear that among the polymorphic loci, RH-specificity is most common: for 14 loci, RH appears to possess an allele that is completely distinct from that possessed by P and C which are closely similar to each other. This was expected based on previous analyses of fewer loci, with fewer enzymes but with many more strains: virulent strains are a clearly distinct (and homogeneous) group compared with nonvirulent strains [Sibley and Boothroyd, 1992].

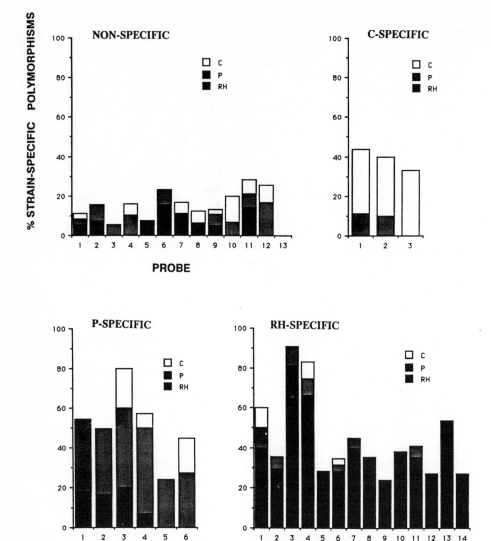

Figure 1. Analysis of polymorphic loci in RH, C and P strains. DNA from each strain was analyzed by restriction enzyme digestion, Southern blotting and probing with each of 36 distinct probes. The results are expressed as vertically stacked histograms showing the percentage of strain-specific polymorphisms (see text) for each of the three strains. The average number of different enzyme digests examined for each probe was 11. The probes have been divided into four groups according to whether there is little polymorphism ("nonspecific"), or according to the strain possessing the allele clearly different from the other two ("C-", "P-" and "RH-specific", respectively).

What was not predicted by the previous study was the existence of C- and P-specific loci where RH bears the same or similar allele as one or other of the two nonvirulent strains. There are at least three possible explanations for their existence. First, and least likely, there could be horizontal gene flow such that without mating, genes are transferred from one member of the population to another (e.g., through the mediation of a virus). There is no evidence to suggest this.

Second, there may be continued but infrequent mating between virulent and nonvirulent strains. This would have to be very rare relative to the expansion of the virulent population as it would introduce heterogeneity into that population which is not seen.

Third, and most likely, the emergence and expansion of the virulent line is not an ancient event and the existence of C- and P-specific loci is indicative of simple polymorphism in the total *T. gondii* gene pool. That is, the virulent line has a more or less random sampling of the gene pool and so has some alleles in common with P and some with C. To confirm this possibility, one would need to know the frequency of each allele in the total gene pool through analysis of a large number of nonvirulent strains (analysis of virulent strains should be unnecessary given their essentially uniform genotype, discussed above). One would also need to know more detail on the exact sequences of these various alleles to judge the approximate time that has elapsed since the emergence of the virulent line.

Conclusion

The clear interpretation of these results is that virulent strains of *T. gondii*, as typified by RH, have broken away from the rest of the *T. gondii* population and developed into a clearly separate lineage. Whether they have evolved to the point of no longer being members of the same species cannot be judged as we do not know the frequencies in the total gene pool of the different alleles being examined. It is clear, however, that if speciation has occurred, it must be a relatively recent event as for many loci, the same or similar alleles are present in the virulent line as in nonvirulent strains. It is also clear from the widespread existence of the virulent line that there is little barrier to the dissemination of a successful Toxoplasma strain as would be guessed from its flexible life cycle and lack of dependence on a particular vector or other environmental condition.

ACKNOWLEDGEMENTS

We are grateful to Erica Boroff, Roland Buelow, John Chen, Allen LeBlanc and Ursula Pley who assisted in the characterization of our data. We are also very grateful to Francisco Ayala, Steve Beverley and Michel Tibayrenc for many helpful discussions of our data. This work was supported by the NIH, the John D. and Catherine T. MacArthur Foundation, Merck Sharp and Dohme and the Burroughs Wellcome Fund.

REFERENCES

Sibley LD, Boothroyd JC (1992) Virulent strains of *Toxoplasma gondii* are clonal. Nature (in press).
Sibley LD, LeBlanc A, Pfefferkorn ER, Boothroyd JC (1992) Generation of a restriction fragment length polymorphism linkage map for *Toxoplasma gondii*. (submitted).

STUDY OF GENETIC POLYMORPHISM OF *TOXOPLASMA* *GONDII* THROUGH ISOENZYME ANALYSIS

M.L. Dardé, B. Bouteille, M. Pestre-Alexandre
Service de Parasitologie
Centre hospitalo-universitaire Dupuytren
87042 Limoges Cedex
FRANCE

Genetic polymorphism is a well-known phenomenon in protozoan species. It has been studied for many years in *Leishmania* sp., *Entamoeba histolytica*, *Trypanosoma* sp., and *Plasmodium falciparum*. *Toxoplasma gondii* is one of the last medically important protozoa to be studied. Several aspects of *T. gondii* epidemiology and biology strongly suggested genetic diversity. This parasite has a wide geographical distribution and a considerable host range. Furthermore, differences in parasite behaviour within the same host species could indicate that the species *T. gondii* may be composed of heterogeneous populations. Based on pathogenicity in Swiss mice, 3 main groups of isolates are generally recognised: acute isolates which kill the mice in 5 to 10 days, chronic or non-pathogenic isolates, and subacute isolates killing the mice within a few weeks or months. Similarly, human toxoplasmosis exhibits a wide range of clinical manifestations which can not entirely be explained by the immune status of the host. Nevertheless, because of the influence of host or environmental factors on extrinsic characteristics, there is no certainty that such variability reflects genetic differences between strains.

The recent application of intrinsic criteria have confirmed the polymorphism of *T. gondii*. Antigenic differences between isolates were detected by Ware and Kasper [1987], while genomic differences were explored by means of restriction fragment length polymorphism (RFLP) [Cristina et al 1991], and molecular karyotyping [Sibley and Boothroyd 1992]. Isoenzyme analysis, which examines a large sample of structural genes, is a standard biochemical technique to assess the level of genetic variations in populations and a useful tool for epidemiological studies. This paper presents the results of such analysis and their contribution to the genetics, epidemiology and biology of *T. gondii*.

Isoenzyme analysis was performed on the tachyzoite stage of cloned *T. gondii* isolates. Large quantities of tachyzoites were obtained from cortisone treated Swiss mice inoculated with both *Toxoplasma* and TG180 murine sarcoma

NATO ASI Series, Vol. H 78
Toxoplasmosis
Edited by Judith E. Smith
© Springer-Verlag Berlin Heidelberg 1993

cells. Parasites were purified from host cells by filtration through polycarbonate membrane (3μm) porosity). Isoenzyme analysis was completed following isofocussing on polyacrylamide (PAG) or agarose gels. Fifteen enzymes were selected for routine characterization of isolates [Darde et al. 1988, 1992a]. This number of enzyme systems is generally considered to be a representative sample of the structural genome of a protozoan [Selander et al 1986, Rioux et al 1990]. Thirteen enzymes were tested after isofocussing in PAGs: acid phosphatase EC 3.1.3.2 (ACP), aconitase EC 4.2.1.3, aldolase EC 4.1.2.13, amylase EC 3.2.1.1 (AMY), aspartate aminotransferase EC 2.6.1.1 (ASAT). catalase EC 1.11.1.6, glucose dehydrogenase EC 1.1.1.47, glucose 6-phosphate dehydrogenase EC 1.1.1.49, glucose phosphate isomerase EC 5.3.1.9 (GPI), glutathione reductase EC 1.6.4.2 (GSR), lactate dehydrogenase EC 1.1.1.27, leucine aminopeptidase, and superoxide dismutase EC 1.15.1.1. Two enzymes were tested after isofocussing in agarose gels, pH gradient 4-6.5: phosphoglucomutase EC 2.7.5.1 (PGM), and propionyl esterase (PE). Thirty-seven isolates have been studied. Six of 15 enzyme systems were polymorphic in this sample: ASAT, GPI, AMY, GSR, PE, and ACP (Figure 1). Two isoenzyme patterns (type I and type II) can be described for ASAT, AMY, GSR, PE and ACP and 3 isoenzyme patterns (types I, II, and III) for GPI. The combination of these isoenzyme patterns allowed the characterisation of 5 zymodemes among the 37 *T. gondii* isolates (Table 1).

Table 1. Zymodemes of 37 *T. gondii* isolates

| Zymodeme | Isoenzyme type | | | | | | Number of isolates |
	ASAT	GSR	AMY	GPI	PE	ACP	
1	I	I	I	I	I	I	6
2	II	II	I	I	II	I	21
3	II	II	II	II	I	I	4
4	II	II	I	III	II	I	5
5	II	I	II	I	I	II	1

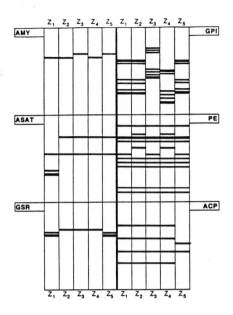

Figure 1. Diagrammatic representation of the isoenzyme patterns of the 6 polymorphic enzymes of the 37 isolates of *T. gondii* clustered into 5 zymodemes (Z1-Z5).

Discussion

Genetic polymorphism of *T. gondii*

The genetic polymorphism detected in our parasite population by this biochemical approach is relatively low. Isoenzyme analysis detected only 5 phenotypes among 37 isolates, that is only a fraction of all possible phenotypes. Over half of the isolates (21 of 37) belong to the same zymodeme, namely Z2. Furthermore, the percentage of common bands between zymodemes, calculated according to the Jaccard similarity coefficient, is high, ranging from 64 to 86%, which indicates no substantial amount of biochemical divergence among *T. gondii* zymodemes. This low polymorphism of *T. gondii* was also suspected by Sibley and Boothroyd [1992] according to the molecular karyotype of 3 isolates. The technique of pulse-field gel electrophoresis (PFGE) detected only 15% variation in migration of chromosomes between strains, far from the widely varying karyotypes seen in *Plasmodium faciparum*. This low diversity is unexpected for *T. gondii* which has a possible sexual life cycle with the consequent genetic exchange systems. This could be explained by the predominance in nature of the asexual cycle, between intermediate hosts and also by the fact that micro and macrogametes are able to fuse and to produce a subsequent progeny. In other words, that selfing is an integral part of *T. gondii* cycle. The consequence at a genetic level is that reduced recombination should be common [Tibayrenc et al 1992].

Epidemiological and biological consequences
Isoenzyme analysis may be applied to large groups of parasites enabling epidemiological studies. When considering geographical aspects, 2 preliminary observations should be made. Firstly, the origins of the isolates are still limited: they originate mainly from various French regions (29 of 37) and only a few have been isolated in the U.S.A. (5 isolates) and in England (3 isolates). Secondly, 25 of the 37 isolates are of human origin and, due to the considerable meat exchange over the world and also to the migration of people, it is difficult to pinpoint the precise geographical origin of human contamination. However, it is notable that the same zymodeme can be found at very distant places (France and California Table 2). Zymodemes do not appear to be site specific, but one could ask if there are different geographical prevalences: Z2 is overrepresented among the French isolates (18 of 29) and 3 of the 5 American isolates studied belong to Z3, which includes only 4 isolates. These differences are not significant, but deserve further investigation involving more isolates originating from different countries.

Table 2 Geographical distribution of zymodemes of 37 *T. gondii* isolates

	Z1	Z2	Z3	Z4	Z5	Total
France	5	18	1	4	1	29
USA	1	1	3	-	-	5
England	-	2	-	1	-	3
	6	21	4	5	1	37

A second epidemiological aspect, the relationship between zymodeme and the original host, is even more difficult to explore because of the large range of possible hosts. In our sample, the range of host species is still limited (Table 3). The isolates originating from human infection predominate (25 of 37) and are found in all the zymodemes. It could be noted that zymodeme 1 includes isolates originating only from human infection.

Table 3. Host origin of the zymodemes of the 37 *T. gondii* isolates

	Z1	Z2	Z3	Z4	Z5	Total
Human	6	13	1	4	1	25
Sheep	-	4	1	-	-	5
Cat	-	2	1	-	-	3
Monkey	-	-	-	1	-	1
Rabbit	-	1	-	-	-	1
Guinea pig	-	-	-	-	-	1
Chicken	-	-	1	-	-	1
	6	21	4	5	1	37

For the present time, the most interesting results of the isoenzyme analysis are the relationships between zymodemes and biological characteristics. This correlation partly confirms the initial hypothesis that biological variability (pathogenicity in mice, oocyst-producing capacity in cats) reflects genetic differences between parasite populations. The most striking evidence is the homogeneous behaviour of the isolates belonging to zyodeme 1. These were all highly pathogenic to mice, such as the well known RH strain, and oocysts could never to obtained for these isolates after feeding cats with brains of mice infected with *Toxoplasma* cysts. Zymodeme 2 contained isolates which were non-pathogenic to mice and for which oocysts were regularly obtained. Zymodemes 3 and 4 included isolates with various degrees of pathogenicity to mice, these were often more pathogenic than Z2 isolates and killed infected mice within a few weeks or months. Oocysts were also regularly obtained from Z3 and Z4 isolates, even for those most pathogenic to mice. Finally, zymodeme 5 contained a single isolate which was highly pathogenic to mice and for which oocyst-producing capacity, studied in only one cat, was absent. More cats need to be infected before any conclusion could be drawn.

Loss of oocyst production can be caused by prolonged and rapid passage of tachyzoites in mice [Frenkel, et al 1976] or in cell culture [Lindsay et al. 1991]. However, one of Z1 isolates was studied for oocyst production after only 4 tachyzoite passages in mice, suggesting that Z1 may be devoid of sexual capacity.

The epidemiological consequences would be that this zymodeme could be maintained in nature solely through intermediate hosts and that this limited cycle would reduce the distribution of Z1 in nature. The validity of this hypothesis must be tested by further epidemiological trials. Molecular and genetic studies are also needed to understand the mechanism of stage-specific regulation in *T. gondii*.

Clinical manifestations.

There was no obvious correlation between zymodeme and the clinical manifestation of human toxoplasmosis (Table 5). If the *T. gondii* strain infecting the patient plays any role in the outcome of the infection, it will be difficult to study as the host immune status plays a major part in the development of this opportunistic parasite.

Table 5. Clinical manifestations associated with the different zymodemes (25 isolates from human origin).

	Z1	Z2	Z3	Z4	Z5	Total
Latent CT*	3	5	1	1	-	10
Severe CT	-	2	-	1	1	4
Aborted CT	2	4	-	1	-	7
Encephalitis	1	1	-	1	-	3
Lymphadenopathies	-	1	-	-	-	1
	6	13	1	4	1	25

*CT: congenital toxoplasmosis

Other Observations

In addition to intraspecific characterization, isoenzyme analysis can provide information on the taxonomic status of related species. *Hammondia hammondi* differs from *T. gondii* by an obligate heterexenous cycle [Frenkel and Dubey, 1975], but is structurally and antigenically very similar [Sheffield et al. 1976, Araujo et al. 1984]. The two parasites have similar $G+C$ content and their ribosomal RNA genes have identical restriction patterns of [Johnson et al. 1987]. Indeed Levine [1977] proposed that *H. hammondi* be considered as a new species of the genus *Toxoplasma*. Isoenzyme analysis of the sporozoite stages of the two parasites allowed a clear distinction between the 2 species. The isoenzyme profiles obtained with the 5 enzyme systems analysed (aconitase, lactate dehydrogenase (LDH), phosphoglucomutase (PGM), ASAT, GPI) for the sporozoites of the 2 species do not share any common bands [Dardé et al. 1992b]. The small number of loci examined do not allow phylogenetic or taxonomic conclusions to be drawn, but do provide new data for further taxonomic discussion.

Host cell specific variations in metabolism

Isoenzyme analysis was usually performed on tachyzoites produced *in vivo* in murine sarcoma cells. When performed with tachyzoites obtained in human fibroblast cell cultures, a new isoenzyme form of LDH appeared for all the isolates [Dardé, et al. 1990a]. This phenotypic variation reflects the adaptability of *T. gondii* to the host cell environment. It could represent one explanation, among others, for the large host range of this parasite.

Stage specific variations in metabolism

Isoenzyme expression in the sporozoite stage of *T. gondii* is lower than in tachyzoites. Many isoenzymes could not be detected after isofocussing of sporozoite extracts. However, some new isoenzyme forms are also present (PGM) and the distinction between the isolates is maintained [Dardé et al. 1990b].

The consequences of the genetic polymorphism of *T. gondii* still cannot be fully evaluated. Genetically different parasite populations with different biological characteristics have been described, but the epidemiological or pathophysiological implications of this polymorphism remain theoretical.

Further studies must be completed using more isolates and additional genomic criteria such as RFLP. The study of strain variability would also be facilitated by an international nomenclature for the designation of *T. gondii* isolates, as established for *Leishmania* isolates. It could include the locality of isolation or the laboratory code, the year of isolation and the name of the original host species to facilitate epidemiological studies.

REFERENCES

Araujo F J, Dubey, J P, Remington J S (1984) Antigenic similarities between the coccidian parasites *Toxoplasma gondii* and *Hammondia hammondi*. Protozool, 31: 145-147.

Cristina, N, Oury B, Ambroise-Thomas P, Santoro F. (1991) Restriction fragment length polymorphisms among *Toxoplasma gondii* strains. Parasitol Res. 77: 266-268.

Dardé M L, Bouteille B, Pestre-Alexandre M (1988) Isoenzymic characterization of seven strains of *Toxoplasma gondii* by isoelectrofocusing in polyacrylamide gels. Am J Trop Med Hyg 39: 551-558.

Dardé M L, Bouteille B, Pestre-Alexandre M (1990a) Comparison of isoenzyme profiles of *Toxoplasma gondii* tachyzoites produced under different culture conditions. Parasitol Res 76: 367-371.

Dardé M L, Bouteille B, Pestre-Alexandre M (1990b) Isoenzymes des tachyzoites et des sporozoites de *Toxoplasma gondii*. Bull Soc Fr Parasitol 8 suppl.1: 237.

Dardé M L, Bouteille B, Pestre-Alexandre M (1992a) Isoenzyme analysis of 35 *Toxoplasma gondii* isolates. Biological and epidemiological implications. J Parasitol, in press.

Dardé M L, Riahi H, Bouteille B, Pestre-Alexandre M (1992b) Isoenzyme analysis of *Hammondia hammondi* and *Toxoplasma gondii* sporozoites. J Parasitol, 78: 731-734.

Frenkel J K, Dubey J P, (1975) *Hammondi hammondi* gen. nov., sp. nov., from domestic cats, a new coccidian related to *Toxoplasma* and Sarcocystiarasitenkd 46: 3-12.

Frenkel J K, Dubey J P, Hoff R L (1976) Loss of stages after continuous passage of *Toxoplasma gondii* and *Besnoitia jellisoni*. J Protozool 23: 421-424.

Johnson A M, Illana S, Dubey J P, Dame J B (1987) *Toxoplasma gondii* and *Hammondia hammondi*: DNA comparison using cloned rRNA genes probes. Exp Parasitol 63: 272-278.

Levine N D (1977) Taxonomy of *Toxoplasma*. J Protozool 24: 36-41.

Lindsay D S, Dubey J P, Blagburn B L, Toivo-Kinnucan M (1991). Examination of tissue cyst formation by *Toxoplasma gondii* in cell cultures using bradyzoites, tachyzoites and sporozoites. J Parasitol 77: 126-132.

Rioux J A, Lanotte G, Serres E, Pratlong F, Bastien P, Perieres J (1990) Taxonomy of *Leishmania*. Use of isoenzymes. Suggestions for a new classification. Ann Parasitol Hum Comp 65: 11-125.

Selander R K, Caugnant D A, Ochman H, Musser J M, Gilmour M N, Whittman T S (1986) Methods of multilocus enzyme electrophoresis for bacterial population genetics and systematics. Appl Environ Microbiol 51: 873-884.

Sheffield H G, Melton, M L, Neva F A (1976) Development of *Hammondia hammondi* in cell cultures. Proc Helminth Soc Washington 43: 217-225.

Sibley L D, Boothroyd J C (1992) Construction of a molecular karyotype for *Toxoplasma gondii*. Mol Biochem Parasitol 51: 291-300.

Tibayrenc M, Kjellberg F, Arnaud J, Oury B, Brénière S F, Dardé M L, Ayala F J (1991) Are eukaryotic micoorganisms clonal or sexual? A population genetics vantage. Proc Natnl Acad Sci USA 88: 5129-5133.

Ware P L, Kasper L H (1987) Strain-specific antigens of *Toxoplasma gondii*. Infect Immun 55: 778-783.

EXPRESSION OF APICAL ORGANELLES ANTIGENS BY A *TOXOPLASMA GONDII* GENOMIC LIBRARY

Odile Mercereau-Puijalon, Marie-Noëlle-Fourmaux*
and Jean-Francois Dubremetz*
Unite de Parasitologie Experimentale, Institut Pasteur, 25 rue du Dr Roux,
75015 Paris, France.

Summary

A genomic library of *Toxoplasma gondii* has been constructed in Lambda gt11. The proteins expressed in *E. coli.* were detected with the serum of a chronically infected rabbit. Specific antibodies were affinity-purified on the proteins expressed by the major reacting clones and used to characterize the corresponding *T. gondii* antigens. Most identified proteins were located in apical organelles (rhoptries, micronemes and dense granules). Additional clones encoding organelle antigens were isolated by screening with a serum from a rabbit immunized with a purified subcellular fraction containing apical organelles. An antiserum raised to recombinant Rop 2/3 reacted with a 100 kDa *Plasmodium falciparum* antigen comigrating with RhopH3.

Introduction

Protozoan parasites of the phylum Apicomplexa possess many common characteristics. In particular, they undergo several differentiation events during their life cycle, yielding distinct forms that possess specific morphological, biochemical, physiological and antigenic characteristics. They are, in their vertebrate host, obligate intracellular parasites. The invasive extracellular forms are equipped at the anterior pole with unique organelles involved in invasion of the cell : rhoptries, dense granules (also called microspheres or dense bodies) and micronemes [Mehlhorn, 1988]. Little is known about the role and biochemical functions devoted to the various organelles in invasion and intracellular establishment. Invasion starts with the attachement of the parasite to the cell surface. This step involves recognition of surface molecules

---

* INSERM U42, 369 rue J. Guesde, 59 650 Villeneuve d'Ascq, France.

NATO ASI Series, Vol. H 78
Toxoplasmosis
Edited by Judith E. Smith
© Springer-Verlag Berlin Heidelberg 1993

by the parasite and the specificity differs from one parasite species to another. Apart from the specific recognition of surface molecules, our hypothesis is that some further steps of the invasion process may be common to several genera and that data obtained for one genus could therefore be transposed to others. We are interested in comparing in that regard *Toxoplasma gondii* and *Pasmodium falcium*, two major pathogens of humans.

We have decided, as a first step, to clone the *T. gondii* genes coding for the proteins stored in the apical organelles. For that purpose, a genomic expression library of *T. gondii* has been constructed in Lambda gt11, and clones expressing antigenic determinants have been isolated by screening with a rabbit antiserum raised by infection as well as with the serum of a rabbit immunized with a subcellular fraction containing the apical organelles. Several clones coding for proteins of the apical organelles have been identified.

Materials and Methods

Parasites : The virulent RH [Sabin, 1941] and the chronic 76K [Laugier & Quilici, 1970] strains of *T. gondii* maintained in Vero cells and in mice, and the *P. falciparum* Palo Alto strain (FUP/CB line) maintained in culture in A+ human red blood cells [Mattei et al, 1988] have been used in this study.

Antibody production : Anti *Toxoplasma* immune serum was obtained from a rabbit that had been infected first with 2000 cysts of strain 76K followed 2 months and 5 months later by 10 000 RH tachyzoites. Anti organelle immune serum was obtained from a rabbit immunized with 3 x 200 ug of a rhoptry-dense granules fraction prepared as described by Leriche & Dubremetz [1991].

Preparation of genomic DNA : 1.5×10^9 parasites (RH strain) were purified from contaminating mouse cells by filtration through polycarbonate filters [Grimwood et al. 1979]. DNA was extracted and purified on Cesium chloride gradients according to Johnson et al. [1986]. The contamination of *T. gondii* DNA with mouse DNA was estimated by using serial dilutions of DNA spotted onto nitrocellulose filters that were hybridized with nick-translated mouse DNA. 25ng of the parasite DNA preparation yielded the same signal as 380pg of pure mouse DNA, indicating that the preparation contained 1-2% of mouse DNA. Before centrifugation, the contamination was about 8%.

Construction and screening of a genomic library : *T. gondii* genomic DNA was prepared from DNAase I-digested essentially as described in Mattei et al. [1988], except that the DNA was also treated with Eco RI methylase. The inserts to be ligated with Lambda gt11 were size-fractionated on a 0.8% agarose gel. The fraction used here was that containing 2Kb-0.5Kb fragments electroeluted from the gel.

For immunological screening, 4,105 phages were plated on Y1090 bacteria, transferred to nitrocellulose filters and probed with the anti-*Toxoplasma* rabbit antiserum, followed by anti-rabbit IgG conjugated with alkaline phosphatase (Promega Biotec). 174 positive lytic plaques were obtained. The plaques yielding strong signals were further grown and purified. The 174 plaques were subjected to a secondary screening using the anti-organelle antiserum, which reacted with 8 clones that were further purified.

Affinity purification of antibodies and characterization of the antigen : Pure bacteriophage clones were spread on agar to express the recombinant proteins on nitrocellulose filters. The antibodies bound to the filters were eluted with 3 M KSCN pH 5.5, immediately dialysed against TBS, and used as such or concentrated 10 times with centricon 30. Immunoblots, immunofluorescence (IFA) and immunoelectromicroscopy using RH tachyzoites were completed as described in Achbarou et al. [1991a].

Analysis of recombinant clones : Lysogens were prepared in *E. coli* Y1089 and bacteriophage production was induced by thermoinduction. DNA was prepared and inserts were recovered by Eco RI digestion and recloned into Eco RI digested pUC13, M13 mp18 (Pharmacia), and pMS 1 vectors [Scherf et al. 1990]. Recombinant B-galactosidases were isolated by affinity chromatography on APTG-sepharose and used to immunise rabbits (100 ug per dose in FCA). Sequencing was done using Sequanase 2. Southern blotting was done as described in Mattei et al [1988]. Some bacteriophage DNAs were hybridized with an insert from the plasmid encoding ROP 1, kindly provided by John Boothroyd [Ossorio et al. 1992].

Results

About 400,000 recombinant phages (about 4 genome equivalents) from the library constructed using fragments in a size range of 500 bp-2000 bp were screened using a rabbit hyperimmune antiserum from an infected animal. The total number of positive clones was 174. Antibodies were affinity-purified on the 44 strongest reacting plaques and used to identify the corresponding parasite antigen by probing immunoblots of RH tachyzoites. The antigen was localized by immunofluorescence on fixed tachyzoites and, when possible, immuno-electron microscopy. Antibodies purified on 13 clones did not produce any signal on immunoblots of tachyzoites, although the specific signal on the recombinant antigen was not lost. The antibodies affinity-purified on 16 clones reacted on immunoblots but the antigen could not be localized. The results of the 15 clones that reacted both on blots and IFA are summarized in Table IA. This collection contains clones encoding rhoptry, microneme and dense granule antigens, as well as one antigen with a typical membrane image. All 174 clones were probed with an anti-organelle rabbit antiserum in order to improve the signals detected and to isolate new specificities. 8 additional clones encoding apical antigens could be isolated. These are indicated in Table IB.

Several clones were studied in more detail for production of recombinant protein and for sizing the *T. gondii* insert. The data are listed in Table I. Most of the strongly reacting clones were producing a ß-galactosidase fusion protein. The signals obtained however were not directly proportional to the amount of protein produced, reflecting different antibody titers and affinity/avidity to the various parasite antigens in the polyspecific serum used. The size of the DNA insert varied from 700 bp to 3000 bp, in the range of the size-fractionated material introduced into the vector.

Rhoptry antigens : Several distinct types of clones encoding rhoptry antigens were obtained. Clones 5.1 and 14.1 cross-reacted. The 14.1 insert hybridized to a plasmid containing ROP 1 sequence, indicating that they are fragments of the ROP 1 gene, encoding the Penetration Enhancing Factor (Ossorio et al. 1992). 23.1 and 44.1 also cross-reacted and cross-hybridized. They are

	PHAGE	FUSION SIZE	INSERT SIZE	PARASITE MW	ANTIGEN LOCALIZATION	IDENTIFIED NAME	REMARKS
A							
	4.1		NT	28	pellicle		id. 32.1
	5.1	no fusion	700	60	Rhoptries	ROP 1	PEF
	5.10	155	NT	40-41	dense granules	GRA 4	id. 36.1 & 37.4
	14.1	180	850	60	Rhoptries	ROP 1	PEF
	16.1	150	1000	20	pellicle		id. 38.1; Mab T4 3G11
	20.1	145	NT	120	Apex	MIC 2	Mab T3 4A11
	23.1	160	1250	55+59	Rhoptries	ROP 2	Tg34; id 44.1
	32.1		NT	28	pellicle		id. 4.1
	34.1		NT				Mab T3 4A7*
	36.1	155	800	40+41	dense granules	GRA 4	id. 5.1 & 37.4
	37.4	155	800	40+41	dense granules	GRA 4	id. 5.1 & 36.1
	38.1	180	800	20	pellicle		id. 16.1; Mab T4 3G11
	42.1	145	800	80,50,48,30	Micronemes	MIC 1	id. 49.1
	44.1	160	1300	55+59	Rhoptries	ROP 2	Tg34; id. 23.1
	49.1	150	1200	80,50,48,30	Micronemes	MIC 1	id. 42.1
B							
	10.3	160	2000	42	Rhoptries	ROP 6	Mab T5 3H12
	24.3	125	700	57-60	Rhoptries	ROP 7?	Mab T4 3H1?
	24.5	125	1000	57-60	Rhoptries	ROP 7?	Mab T4 3H1?
	26.3	123	1700	> 200	Rhoptries?	ROP 8?	
	30.1	140	800	59.5	Rhoptries?	ROP 5?	Mab T5 3E2
	40.3	160	1600	42	Rhoptries	ROP 6	Mab T5 3H12
	40.5		1500	42	Rhoptries	ROP 6	Mab T5 3H12
	46.3		900	28	dense granules	GRA 2	Mab T4 1F5

Table 1: List of the clones isolated by screening using an anti *Toxoplasma* rabbit antiserum (A) and reacting strongly with an anti rhoptry/dense granule antiserum (B). The size of the fusion protein and of the parasite antigen are in kDa, and that of the DNA insert is expressed in bp. id indicates a sibling clone. *clone 34.1 reacted with Mab T3 4A7, which defines a rhoptry protein of 60 kDa. PEF and references thereof are described in Ossorio et al. [1992]. Mabs T4 3G11 is described in Couvreur et al. 1988], Mab T3 4A11 in Achbarou et al. [1991a], mab T5 3H12, T4 3H1, T5 3E2 in Leirche & Dubremetz [1991] and Mab T4 1F5 in Achbarou et al [1991b]. the correspondence of these antigens with those described in the literature is discussed in the references cited.

derived from the same gene, encoding a 55-59 kDa rhoptry antigen previously described as ROP2-ROP3 [Leriche & Dubremetz, 1991] and reacted with Mab T4 2F8, specific for these proteins [Sadak et al, 1988]. Clone 34.1 reacted

reacted with Mab T3 4A7, indicating that it may encode the 60kDa rhoptry antigen ROP 4 [Leriche & Dubremetz, 1991]. This latter clone has not yet been studied in detail and its precise identification needs to be verified.

Four other types of clones were obtained by the secondary screening using an antiserum raised to the organelle subcellular fraction, as listed in Table IB. For those, the rhoptry localization was determined by IFA and awaits further confirmation by immuno EM. 10.3, 40.3 and 40.5 were specific for a 42 kDa molecule comigrating with ROP6.

Antibodies purified on 24.3 and 24.5 reacted with a protein doublet of 57-60 kDa : the 57 kDa comigrated with a band identified by Mab T4 3H1 [Leriche & Dubremetz, 1991] and has been tentatively named ROP 7, whereas the 60 kDa protein comigrated with ROP 4, however its possible identity with ROP 4 awaits confirmation. Antibodies purified on 26.3 were specific for a rhoptry antigen migrating as several high molecular weight bands over 200 kDa, which has been tentatively named ROP 8. Finally, 30.1 enabled purification of antibodies that reacted with an antigen comigrating with ROP 5 at 59.5 kDa.

Micronemes : Two clones, 42.1 and 49.1, yielded the same specificity : a 60 kDa protein. The antigen was located by immunoelectronmicroscopy in micronemes. This antigen was called MIC 1 [Achbarou et al. 1991a]. Antibodies purified on clone 20.1 reacted with a 120 kDa antigen comigrating with MIC 2 defined by Mab T3 4A11 [Achbarou et al. 1991a], and produced an apical fluorescence. 20.1 is thus likely to be specific for MIC2.

Dense granules : Several clones were used to affinity-purify antibodies reacting with dense granules. 5.10, 36.1 and 37.4 were sibling clones derived from a gene encoding a new dense granule antigen, GRA 4, that is described in detail elsewhere [Mévélec, et al. submitted]. Antibodies affinity-purified on 46.3 reacted with a band that comigrated with Mab T4 1F5, and produced the same image. This indicated that this clone is probably part of the GRA 2 gene [Achbarou et al. 1991b].

Other apical and membrane antigens : Antibodies affinity-purified on clones 4.1 and 32.1 cross reacted and recognized a 28 kDa membrane antigen. Clone 16.1 identified a 20 kDa membrane antigen.

Cross-reaction of 23.1 with P. falciparum : Clone 23.1 was studied in detail. The insert from clone 23.1 was used to probe RH genomic DNA in Southern blots, as shown in Fig 1. Two bands hybridized with the probe after digestion with several enzymes for which no sites exist within the insert. Under stringent conditions, the strong signal was maintained, whereas the fainter one was lost (data not shown). This indicates the existence of a duplicated sequence homologous to 23.1.

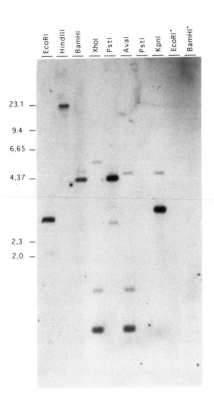

Figure 1: Southern blot of tachyzoite DNA probed with the 23.1 insert. The restriction enzymes used are listed on top of each lane. The lanes on the right marked with an asterik were loaded with mouse DNA digested as indicated. On the left is indicated the migration of the markers (in Kb).

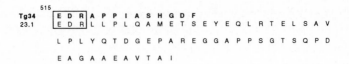

```
          515
Tg34      E D R A P P I A S H G D F
23.1      E D R L L P L Q A M E T S E Y E Q L R T E L S A V

          L P L Y Q T D G E P A R E G G A P P S G T S Q P D

          E A G A A E A V T A I
```

Figure 2: Predicted protein sequence of 23.1 (bottom) compared with that of Tg34. The sequence shown was translated downstream from amino acid 515 of TG34. The frame shift occurs just after the Arg codon.

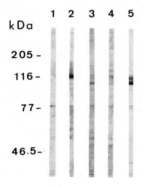

Figure 3: Immunoblot of *P. falciparum* probed with an antiserum raised to the 254 β-galactosidase expressing the 23.1 insert (lane 2: preimmune serum : lane 1), with anti 249 β-galactosidase expressing the 14.1 insert (lane 4; preimmune serum : lane 3) and with anti Ag44 β-galactosidase expressing the C-terminal region of RhopH3 (lane 5).

DNA sequencing showed that the 23.1 insert was almost identical to the 3' end of the gene Tg34 described by Saavedra et al. [1991]. The 23.1 sequence starts at position 547 of the Tg34 sequence and ends at the same point, a genuine Eco RI site of *T. gondii* DNA. A few differences were observed. At nucleotides 1171-1172 a GC was observed instead of a CG, resulting in two amino acid changes (HV instead of QL). At nucleotide 1589-1591, instead of a GGG present in Tg34, we observed in 4 different templates a GG, and this was confirmed using dITP. This modifies the subsequent reading frame, as shown in Fig 2.

The last difference was at position 1690 a C instead of a T. Fig 3 shows that antibodies raised to ß-galactosidase 254 (i.e. the 23.1 insert fused to the ß-galactosidase of vector pMS 1) reacted with *P. falciparum* on immunoblot, recognizing a 100 kDa band (lane 2). This is comigrating with the upper band of a rhoptry antigen called RhopH3 [Lustigman et al, 1988] (lane 5). Anti ß-galactosidase 249 (containing the 14.1 insert encoding part of ROP 1) did not react significantly on this blot (lane 4) nor did preimmune rabbit sera (lanes 1 and 3, respectively).

Discussion

The approach reported here enabled the isolation of numerous clones expressing *T. gondii* antigens, most of which localized in the exocytic apical organelles. Two as yet undescribed apical antigens, MIC 1 and GRA 4 were identified. It is interesting to note that all the antigens analysed in this work had migration properties in SDS PAGE not significantly altered by prior treatment with DTT, indicating that they contain few if any disulphide bridges. Antibodies purified on several clones produced specific and unambiguous signals on immunoblots of tachyzoites but were negative in IFA, indicating that the parasite antigen is either masked within a complex, or folded differently in the preparations used for immunolocalization.

The relatively large number of sibling clones collected from distinct Petri dishes was unexpected, as the number of genome equivalents screened was not large. It is possible that only a fraction of the *T. gondii* antigens are mimicked in a bacterial expression system. Another reason is that some fragments are overrepresented. In most cases analysed so far, the DNA inserts of the sibling clones end in 3' at a natural Eco RI site. This indicates that the methylation step performed during the construction of the library in order to protect endogenous Eco RI sites was incomplete, resulting in a relative enrichment in certain Eco RI fragments and favouring their subsequent cloning. Antibodies affinity-purified on one third of the clones failed to identify the corresponding antigen, despite the fact that the antibody preparation was still able to bind to the recombinant antigen. We suspect that this group of clones may contain genes encoding antigens expressed at another life stage, possibly bradyzoites. The rabbit serum used to screen the library was collected from an animal injected with 76K cysts, and some of the antibodies produced may be specific for bradyzoite antigens. This possibility is being explored and is not unlikely, as the library used here was a genomic library, containing the information for all life stages and for all developmental steps.

One of the clones isolated, 23.1, encodes a rhoptry antigen of 55-59 kDa. DNA sequencing indicated that 23.1 was part of gene Tg 34, described recently by Saavedra et al. [1991]. Our sequence differs from that of Tg 34 in one major point, resulting in a frame-shift in the region encoding the C-terminus. Whether this reflects genetic polymorphism in that region or a cloning artefact remains to be clarified: in particular antibodies to the C-terminal region will be raised. The 23.1 protein reacted strongly with Mab T4 2F8, which labels the rhoptries and reacts with a 66 kDa major and a 71 kDa minor antigen chased into a 55 kDa major and a 59 kDa minor polypeptide [Sadak et al. 1988]. Consistent with this, an antiserum raised to the recombinant β-galactosidase 254 containing the 23.1 insert reacted strongly with the body of the rhoptries and, on immunoblots, recognised 2 bands of 59 and 55 kDa. The 55 and 59 kDa proteins were named ROP 2 & 3 respectively by Leriche & Dubremetz [1991]. Our data indicate that the 23.1/Tg34 gene codes for these proteins. As the exact relationship between both antigens is unclear, we tentatively call this gene ROP 2/3. We still need to determine whether the 55kDa and the 59 kDa antigens are encoded by distinct genes or are different processing products of the same gene. Interestingly, Southern blotting using the 23.1 probe showed the existence of a related gene. This cross-hybridizing gene may code for the 59 kDa antigen. Alternatively, it may be the gene for the third band of the T3 4A7 complex, a 60 kDa protein named ROP 4 by Leriche & Dubremetz [1991], shown to share antigenic determinants with the 55 kDa and the 59 kDa antigens [Sadak et al. 1988]. The fact that the gene is duplicated is reminiscent of other genes coding for antigens of the apical pole in Apicomplexa, such as the Duffy receptor of *P. knowlesi*, located in the micronemes [Adams et al. 1990] or the 235 kDa rhoptry protein of *P. yoelii* [Keen et al. 1990]. These genes are present in several copies in the genome, constituting families coding for proteins involved in recognition of the surface of the target cell.

Some monoclonal antibodies have been reported to react with distinct genera of the phylum Apicomplexa [Taylor et al, 1990; Suarez et al, 1991], arguing in favour of conserved structures (and functions ?). Apart from the C-terminus which differs in RH and Wiktor strains, the ROP 2/3 antigen is well conserved in *T. gondii*, and immunological cross-reaction with *P. falciparum* indicates the presence of a related antigen in *Plasmodia*. In *P. falciparum*, the anti β-galactosidase 254 antibodies reacted with a band at about 100kDa. Interestingly, the only significant homology, observed with antigens of *P. falciparum* migrating at 100 kDa, to date is with two short sequences of a rhoptry antigen, RhopH3 [Brown and Coppel, 1991]. This cross reaction will be investigated using synthetic peptides. It would be interesting to determine whether this homology has a functional significance and could be extended to other apical organelle proteins.

References

Achbarou A., Mercereau-Puijalon O., Autheman J.M., Fortier B., Camus D, Dubremetz J.F. (1991a)   Characterization of microneme proteins of microneme proteins of *Toxoplasma gondii*.   Mol Biochem Parasitol 47 : 223-234.

Achbarou A, Mercereau-Puijalon O., Sadak A., Fortier B., Leriche M.A. Camus D. proteinsin the parasitophorous vacuole of *Toxoplasma gondii*. Parasitology 103 : 321-329.

Adams J.H., Hudson D.E., Torii M., Ward G.E., Wellems T.E., Aikawa M., Miller L.H. (1990).   The Duffy receptor family of *Plasmodium knowlesi* is located within the micronemes of invasive malaria merozoites. Cell 63 : 141-153.

Brown H.J. & Coppel R.L. (1991)   Primary structure of a *Plasmodium falciparum* rhoptry antigen. Mol Biochem Parasitol 49 : 99-110.

Couvreur G, Sadak A., Fortier B., Dubremetz J.F. (1988)   surface antigens of *Toxoplasma gondii* : Parasitology, 97 : 1-10.

Grimwood B.G., Hechemy K., Stevens R.W. (1979)   *Toxoplasma gondii:* Purification of trophozoites propagated in cell culture.   Exp Parasitol 48 : 282-286.

Johnson A.M., Dubey J.P., Dame J.B. (1986) Purification and characterization of *Toxoplasma gondii* : tachyzoite DNA. Aust J Exp Biol Med Sci 64 : 351-355.

Keen J., Holder A.A., Playfair J., Lockyer M., Lewis A (1990) Identification of the gene for a *Plasmodium yoelii* rhoptry protein. Multiple copies in the parasite genome. Mol Biochem Parasitol 42 : 241-246.

Laugier M & Quilici M.(1970) Intérêt expérimental d'une souche de Toxoplasme peu pathogène pour la souris. Ann Parasitol Hum Comp 45 : 389-403.

Leriche M.A., & Dubremetz J.F. (1991) Characterization of the protein contents of rhoptries and dense granules of *Toxoplasma gondii* tachyzoites by subcellular fractionation and monoclonal antibodies. Mol Biochem Parasitol 45 : 249-260.

Lustigman S., Anders R.F., Brown G.V. & Coppel R.L. (1988) A component of an antigenic rhoptry complex of *Plasmodium falciparum* is modified after merozoite invasion. Mol Biochem Parasitol 30, 217-224.

Mattei D., Langsley G., Braun-Breton C., Guillotte M., Dubremetz J.F., Mercereau-Puijalon O (1988) The S-antigen of *Plasmodium falciparum* Palo Alto represents a new S-antigen serotype. Mol Biochem Parasitol 27 : 171-180.

Mehlhorn H (1988) Cellular organization of the Protozoa. In Parasitology in Focus, Mehlhorn H (ed), Springer Verlag, pp161-188.

Ossorio P.N., Schwartzman J.D., Boothroyd J.C. (1992) A *Toxoplasma gondii* rhoptry protein associated with host cell penetration has unusual charge asymmetry. Mol Biochem Parasitol 50 : 1-16.

Saavedra R., De Meuter F., Decourt J.L., Hérion P (1991) Human T cell clone identifies a potentially protective 54-kDa protein antigen of *Toxoplasma gondii* cloned and expressed in *Escherichia coli.* J Immunol 147 : 1975-1982.

Sabin A.B. (1941) Toxoplasmic encephalitis in children. J Am Med Assoc 116 : 801-807.

Sadak A., Taghy Z., Fortier B., Dubremetz J.F., (1988) Characterization of a family of rhoptry proteins of *Toxoplasma gondii.* Mol Biochem Parasitol 29 : 203-211.

Scherf A., Mattei D, Schreiber M (1990) Parasite antigens expressed in *Escherichia coli.* A refined approach for epidemiological analysis. J Immunol Methods 128 : 81-87.

Suarez C.E., McElwain T.F., Stephens E.B., Mishra V.A., Palmer G.H., (1991) Sequence conversation among merozoite apical complex proteins of *Babesia bovis, Babesia bigemina* and other Apicomplexa. Mol Biochem Parasitol 49 : 329-332.

Taylor D.W., Evans C.B., Aley S.A., Barta J., Danforth H.D. (1990) Identification of an apically-located antigen that is conserved in sporozoan parasites. J. Protozool 37 : 540-545.

DENSE GRANULE ANTIGENS OF *TOXOPLASMA GONDII*

M-F. CESBRON-DELAUW*, C. MERCIER*, L. LECORDIER*, F. DARCY*$ AND
A. CAPRON*

* Centre d'Immunologie et de Biologie Parasitaire
INSERM 624 - CNRS 167
Institut Pasteur de Lille
1 rue du Professeur A. Calmette
59045 LILLE
FRANCE

In the search for protective antigens aiming at the development of a sub-unit vaccine against toxoplasmosis, several molecules have been found to represent good candidates, in particular P30 or SAG1, the major surface antigen of tachyzoite [Burg et al., 1988; Bülow and Boothroyd, 1991]. In contrast, previous work in our laboratory has highlighted the great interest of tachyzoite excreted-secreted antigens (ESAs) for a vaccine [Darcy et al., 1988; Decoster et al., 1988; Ridel et al., 1988 ; Duquesne et al., 1990; Darcy et al., 1992]. These ESAs have been found to be stored in the dense granules of *Toxoplasma gondii*.

Their secretion into the parasitophorous vacuole that occurs after host-cell invasion suggests a role in the survival of the parasite within the host-cell. Furthermore, they have been reported

- to be immunogenic during human and experimental infections [Darcy et al., 1988 ; Decoster et al., 1988];

$ Present address : CHR ANGERS, 4 Rue de Larrey, 49033 ANGERS
FRANCE

NATO ASI Series, Vol. H 78
Toxoplasmosis
Edited by Judith E. Smith
© Springer-Verlag Berlin Heidelberg 1993

- to protect highly susceptible nu/nu rats, inducing both antibody-dependent [Darcy et al., 1988] and cellular [Ridel et al., 1988; Duquesne et al., 1990] immune responses ;

- to protect mice orally infected by a lethal dose of tachyzoites [Darcy et al., 1992].

Some of these ESAs have been identified to share common epitopes with antigens of bradyzoites [Darcy et al., 1990]. These antigens might provide a molecular basis for the mechanism of concomitant immunity [Capron and Dessaint, 1988] and have thus been chosen in our laboratory as candidates for the development of a vaccine.

The production of ESAs from tachyzoites in cell-free medium containing 10% of serum [Darcy et al., 1988] and the production of monoclonal antibodies (mAbs) [Charif et al., 1990] led us to characterize some of these antigens at the molecular level.

The use of the mAbs in immunogold labeling has clearly demonstrated the storage of 3 ESAs [P23, GP28.5, and P21] in the dense granules of *T. gondii* [Cesbron-Delauw et al., 1989; Charif et al., 1990]. These 3 antigens have been further referred as GRA1 (P23), GRA2 (GP28.5) and GRA5 (P21), following the nomenclature of Sibley et al. [1991]. Two other GRA molecules have also been localized in the dense granules, a GRA3 of 30 kDa [Achbarou et al., 1991] and a GRA4 of 40 kDa [Achbarou et al., 1991; Mevelec et al., 1992]. The 5 GRA antigens described up to now present the common feature of being released from the dense granules into the parasitophorous vacuole after host-cell invasion [Sibley and Sharma, 1987; Cesbron-Delauw et al., 1989; Charif et al., 1990; Achbarou et al., 1991; Lecordier et al., submitted]. However, these 5 antigens have been shown to be differentially targetted in the parasitophorous vacuole, the GRA1, GRA2 and GRA4 molecules being found in vacuolar space, preferentially associated with the tubular network, whereas the GRA3 and GRA5 are associated with the vacuole membrane [Cesbron-Delauw et al., 1989; Charif et al., 1990; Achbarou et al., 1991].

Furthermore, some B and T-cell epitopes have been characterized within the GRA1 and GRA2 molecules. Indeed, among the synthetic peptides derived from the GRA1 sequence, two C-terminal peptides (170-193 and 194-208) have been identified as T-cell epitopes, whilst the former is also a B-cell epitope recognized by the mouse anti-GRA1 mAb TG17-43 (Duquesne et al., 1991). Serological studies using human sera and truncated recombinant GRA2 have shown that this antigen contains at least 3 B epitopes [Murray et al., in preparation]. One of them, the C-terminal, is recognized by the mouse anti-GRA2 mAb TG17-179 and is probably linear [Cesbron-Delauw et al., 1992].

MOLECULAR CHARACTERIZATION OF GRA1, GRA2 AND GRA5

GRA genes organization

Molecular cloning of the genes encoding the GRA1, GRA2 and GRA5 molecules was also carried out in order to provide the molecular tools to investigate firstly, their function in the host-parasite interaction [Cesbron-Delauw et al., 1989; Cesbron-Delauw et al., 1992; Mercier et al., in press; Lecordier et al., submitted] and secondly, their gene regulation. Indeed, their storage in the same subcellular compartment allows to envisage common regulatory signals for their expression.

Comparison of the cDNA and genomic sequences led us to deduce some common features amongst the 3 GRA genes, which are probably present in the Toxoplasma genome as a single copy.

- The transcription start site does not seem to depend on the presence of traditional signals like TATA- and/or CAAT-boxes. In contrast, GC-rich sequences which could serve as these signals were found in the 250 bp region upstream of the cap site. The same observation can be made for other cloned T. gondii genes [SAG1 : Burg et al., 1988; α- and β-tubulins : Nagel & Boothroyd., 1988; ROP1 : Ossorio et al., 1992)]

- Several T-stretches are present upstream of the ATG initiation codon in the 5' untranslated sequence. These motifs are observed in the two regions bordering the cap site when compared with other genes of T. gondii .

- A rather long 3' untranslated sequence is present in the 3 genes.

Among the 5 GRA genes cloned up to now, only the GRA2 one contains an intron in the coding sequence. The 5'- and 3'-splice junctions of this intron show high homology with the consensus boundary sequences.

On the basis of DNA sequences and subcellular distribution, GRA2 [Mercier et al., in press] appeared to be identical to the protective antigen of 28 kDa described by Sibley and Sharma [Sharma et al., 1984; Sibley and Sharma, 1987], cloned by Prince et al. [Prince et al., 1989] and corrected by Parmley et al. [Parmley et al. in press].

Characteristics of the amino acid sequences of the GRA proteins

Comparison of the GRA1 [Cesbron-Delauw et al., 1989], GRA2 [Cesbron-Delauw et al., 1992 ; Mercier et al., in press] and GRA5 [Lecordier et al.,

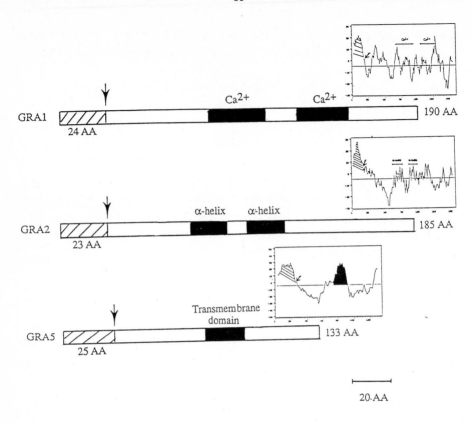

Fig. 1 : Schematic representation of the deduced amino acid structure of GRA1, GRA2 and GRA5, including hydrophobic profiles. The putative signal peptides are shaded. The arrows show the probable cleavage site of signal peptides. Black boxes represent the predicted calcium binding domain (EF-hand) of GRA1, the predicted amphiphatic α-helices of GRA2 and the predicted transmembrane domain of GRA5. The plots of hydrophobicity were determined by the Kyte and Doolittle method [Kyte and Doolittle, 1982]. The segment length for analysis was 9 amino acids. The horizontal axes show the amino acid number along the protein. The vertical axes show the units of hydropathicity as calculated by the algorithm, with a maximum of 30 for GRA1 and GRA2 and a maximum of 50 for GRA5.

submitted] amino acid sequences (Fig. 1) provides many interesting pieces of information about their maturation, their folding and their targeting.

- The presence of a typical signal peptide targeting the proteins to the secretory pathway can be deduced from the primary structure analysis of the 3 GRA proteins.

- Some post-translational modifications are envisaged for the 3 antigens :

i)- a modification of the N-terminal amino acid, since no N-terminal sequence could be obtained by the Edman degradation method [Edman and Begg, 1967] after HPLC purification of the native antigens. In contrast, several peptides covering the entire mature polypeptide deduced from the cDNA were found after partial degradation of the native purified antigens.

ii)- O-glycosylation(s), because of the presence of many serine and threonine residues in the 3 amino acid sequences.

The analysis of the amino acid sequences of GRA1, GRA2 and GRA5 reveals a clear distribution of the hydrophobic and hydrophilic residues. Except for the first N-terminal region corresponding to the signal peptide, a second domain, different for each GRA polypeptide, may be related to their distribution in the parasitophorous vacuole.

- The presence of two calcium binding domains characterized by an α-helix-loop-α-helix structure, known as EF-hand, has been predicted in the GRA1 sequence. The Ca^{2+}-binding property of the recombinant and native antigens (Cesbron-Delauw et al., 1989; Charif et al., 1990) has been demonstrated. GRA1, which is detected in the matrix of the parasitophorous vacuole, may thus function as a Ca^{2+} buffer modulating the Ca^{2+}-concentration to stabilize the network of the parasitophorous vacuole.

- The hydrophobic and hydrophilic residues of the central region of GRA2 could be separated in two repeated domains arranged as two amphiphatic α-helices. The length of the helices would be sufficient to ensure transmembrane spanning domains which could form a pore through the tubulomembranous structures of the network, in the condition of (homo- or hetero-) polymerization of GRA2. Alternatively, the two amphiphatic α-helices could be arranged in an antiparallel framework, in which the hydrophobic surfaces would be buried inside the molecule while the hydrophilic residues would be located on the surface, ensuring an electrostatical binding of GRA2 to membranes. Such association with membranes is observed for amphitropic proteins which are soluble in water and interact with phospholipids of membranes in a calcium-dependent manner [Burn, 1988]. This is in agreement with the observations of Sibley and Boothroyd [1992] that Ca^{2+}-regulated secretion of the GRA2 protein occurs with both soluble and membranous forms. In addition, some amphitropic proteins have been reported to interact with EF-hand proteins [Gerke, 1991], suggesting a possible association of GRA2 with GRA1 whose calcium buffer role may stabilize the interaction of GRA2 with membranous structures of the network.

- In contrast, the second and central hydrophobic domain of GRA5 displays the characteristics of a typical transmembrane helix. Whether the GRA5 antigen is permanently anchored in the parasitophorous vacuole membrane through its putative transmembrane domain remains to be investigated. However, in agreement with this hypothesis, ultrastructural observations have shown a clear association of GRA5 with the vacuole membrane and recent studies have shown an abundant distribution of this antigen to the more external cystic membrane [Torpier et al., submitted]. The presence of a secreted protein of *Toxoplasma gondii* in vacuole or cyst membranes suggests that these membranes are either synthetized by the parasites or strongly modified by the parasite molecules.

In conclusion, although the exact role of the GRA molecules in parasite-host-cell interaction remains to be defined, the molecular characterization of the GRA proteins has allowed us to propose a functional (Ca^{2+}-dependent) association between GRA2 and GRA1, the two major secreted antigens of *Toxoplasma* dense granules. The Ca^{2+}-binding property of GRA1 suggests its physiological importance in the secretion process during cell invasion whereas the particular localization of GRA5 suggests the participation of this molecule in the cyst and paprasitophorous vacuole membrane functions.

Acknowledgements.
The authors are particularly grateful to D. Deslée and to M-P. Fourmaux for their excellent technical assistance.

References.
Achbarou, A., Mercereau-Puijalon, O., Sadak, A., Fortier, B., Leriche, M.A., Camus, D., and Dubremetz, J.F. (1991) Differential targeting of dense granule proteins in the parasitophorous vacuole of *Toxoplasma gondii*. Parasitol. 103: 321-329

Büllow, R. and Boothroyd, J.C. [1991] Protection of mice from fatal *Toxoplasma gondii* infection by immunization with P30 antigen in liposomes. J. Immunol. 147: 3496-3500.

Burg, J.L., Perelman, D., Kasper, L., Ware, P.L., and Boothroyd, J.C. [1988] Molecular analysis of the gene encoding the major surface antigen of *Toxoplasma gondii*. J. Immunol. 141: 3584-3591.

Burn, B. [1988] Amphitropic proteins : a new class of membrane proteins. TIBS 13: 79-83.

Capron, A. and Dessaint, J.P. [1988] Vaccination against parasitic diseases : some alternative concepts for the definition of protective antigens. Ann. Inst. Past./Immunol. 139: 109-117.

Cesbron-Delauw, M.F., Guy, B., Torpier, G., Pierce, R.J., Lenzen, G., Cesbron, J.Y., Charif, H., Lepage, P., Darcy, F., Lecocq, J.P., and Capron, A. [1989] Molecular characterization of a 23-KDa major antigen secreted by *Toxoplasma gondii*. Proc. Natl. Acad. Sci. USA. 86: 7537-7541.

Cesbron-Delauw, M.F., Boutillon, C., Mercier, C., Fourmaux, M.P Murray, A., Miquey, F., Tartar, A., and Capron, A. [1192] Amino acid sequence requirements for the epitope recognized by a monoclonal antibody reacting with the secreted antigen G.P.28.5 of *Toxoplasma gondii*. Mol. Chem. 29: 1375-1382.

Charif, H., Darcy, F., Torpier, G., Cesbron-Delauw, M.F., and Capron, A. [1990] *Toxoplasma gondii* : Characterization and localization of antigens secreted from tachyzoites. Exp. Parasitol. 71: 114-124.

Darcy, F., Deslée, D., Santoro, F., Charif, H., Auriault, C., Decoster, A., Duquesne, V., and Capron, A. [1988] Induction of a protective antibody-dependent response against toxoplasmosis by in vitro excreted-secreted antigens from tachyzoites of *Toxoplasma gondii*. Parasite Immunol. 10: 553-567.

Darcy, F., Charif, H., Caron, H., Deslée, D. Pierce, R.J., Cesbron-Delauw, M.F., Decoster, A., and Capron, A. [1990] Identification and biochemical characterization of antigens of tachyzoites and brayzoites of *Toxoplasma gondii* with cross-reactive epitopes. Parasitol. Res. 76: 473-478.

Darcy, F., Torpier, G., Cesbron-Delauw, M.F., Decoster, A. and Capron A. [1992] Diagnostic et prévention de la toxoplasmose : nouvelles approches et perspectives. Gynécol. Intern. 1: 48-57.

Decoster, A., Darcy, F., and Capron, A. [1988] Recognition of *Toxoplasma gondii* excreted and secreted antigens by human sera from acquired and congenital toxoplasmosis : identification of markers of acute and chronic infection. Clin. Exp. Immunol. 73: 376-382.

Dusquesne, V., Auriault, C., Darcy, F., Decavel, J.P., and Capron, A. [1990] Protection of nude rats against *Toxoplasma* infection by excreted-secreted antigens [ESA] specific helper T cells. Infect. Immun. 58: 2120-2126.

Dusquesne, V., Auriault, C., Gras-Masse, H., Boutillon, C., Darcy, F., Cesbron-Delauw, M.F., Tartar, A., and Capron, A. [1991] Identification of T-cell epitopes within a 23-kDa antigen (P24) of *Toxoplasma gondii*. Clin. Exp. Immunol. 84: 527-534.

Edman, P., and Begg, G., [1967] A protein sequenator. Eur. J. Biochem. 1: 80-91.

Gerke, V. [1991] p11, a member of the S-100 family, is associated with the tyrosin kinase substrate p36 (AnnexinII) In : Novel calcium binding proteins. Fundamentals and clinical implications. (Heizmann, C.W., ed.) pp 139-155. Springer Verlag.

Kyte, J. and Doolittle R.F. [1982] A simple method for displaying the hydrophobic character of a protein. J. Mol. Biol. 157: 105-132.

Mercier, C., Lecordier, L., Darcy, F., Deslée, D., Murray, A., Tourvieille, B., Maes, P., Capron, A., and Cesbron-Delauw, M.F. (In Press) *Toxoplasma gondii* : molecular characterization of a dense granule antigen (GRA2) associated with the network of the parasitophorous vacuole. Molec. Biochem. Parasitol.

Mevelec, M.N., Chardes, T., Mercereau-Puijalon, O., Bourguin, I., Achbarou, A., Dubremetz, J.F., and Bout, D. [1992] Molecular cloning of GRA4, a *Toxoplasma gondii* dense granule protein recognized by mucosal IgA antibodies. Molec. Biochem. Parasitol. 56 : 227-238.

Nagel, S.D. and Boothroyd, J.C. [1988] The α- and β-tubulins of *Toxoplasma gondii* are encoded by simple copy genes containing multiple introns. Mol. Biochem. Parasitol. 29: 261-273.

Ossorio, P.N., Schwartzman, J.D., and Boothroyd, J.C. [1992] A *Toxoplasma gondii* rhoptry protein associated with host cell penetration has unusual charge asymetry. Mol. Biochem. Parasitol. 50: 1-16.

Parmley, S.F., Sgarlato, G.D. and Remington, J.S. (In Press) Genomic and corrected cDNA sequence of the P28 gene from *Toxoplasma gondii*. Mol. Biochem. Parasitol.

Prince, J.B., Araujo, F.G., Remington, J.S., Burg, L., Boothroyd, J.C., and Sharma, S.D. [1989] Cloning of cDNAs encoding a 28 kilodalton antigen of *Toxoplasma gondii*. Mol. Biochem. Parasitol. 34: 3-14.

Ridel, P.R., Auriault, C., Darcy, F., Pierce, R.J., Leite, P., Santoro, F., Neyrinck, J.L., Kusnierz, J.P., and Capron, A. (1988) Protective role of IgE in immunocompromised rat toxoplasmosis. J. Immunol. 141: 978-983.

Sharma, S.D., Araujo, F.G. and Remington, J.S., [1984] *Toxoplasma* antigen isolated by affinity chromatography with monoclonal antibody protects mice against lethal infection with *Toxoplasma gondii*. J. Immunol. 133: 2818-2820.

Sibley, L.D. and Sharma, S.D. [1987] Ultrastructural localization of an intracellular *Toxoplasma* protein that induces protection in mice. Infect. Immun. 55: 2137-2141.

Sibley, L.D., Pfefferkorn, E.R., and Boothroyd, J.C. [1991] Proposal for a uniform genetic nomenclature in *Toxoplasma gondii*. Parasitol. Today. 7: 327-328.

Sibley, L.D., and Boothroyd, J.C. [1992] Calcium-regulated secretion and modification of host-cell endocytic compartments by *Toxoplasma*. Abstract in J. Cell Biochem. Suppl. 16A : 163.

A STRATEGY FOR CLONING A DNA POLYMERASE GENE OF TOXOPLASMA GONDII

A.M. Johnson, A. Makioka and J.T. Ellis
Department of Microbiology
University of Technology, Sydney
Westbourne Street
Gore Hill, New South Wales
Australia 2065

Introduction

Recent research on the molecular biology of *Toxoplasma gondii* has been focused on the isolation and characterisation of genes encoding immunologically important antigens that may form the basis of anti-parasite vaccines [Johnson, 1989; Ellis and Johnson, 1992]. Membrane, rhoptry and secreted antigens have been identified, characterised and cloned [McLeod *et al.*, 1991; Ossorio *et al.*, 1992; Parmley *et al.*, 1992]. However, the biology of DNA replication in coccidian parasites has not been studied using recombinant DNA techniques.

In eukaryotes the process of DNA replication is a complex procedure requiring the co-operation of many enzymes. Eukaryotic cells are known to contain at least three nuclear and one mitochondrial DNA polymerase. The properties of these enzymes have been reviewed and a generalised model for initiation of DNA replication presented [Campbell, 1986; Wang, 1991]. An enzyme complex containing DNA polymerase/DNA primase is central to the formation of the initiation complex, and it therefore has a major regulatory role. Initiation of DNA replication is thought to occur at specific DNA sequences within replicons, known as "origins of replication". Following initiation, fidelity of copying DNA during replication and repair relies on the ability of the DNA polymerases to accurately copy the template strand. Two distinct DNA polymerases, $\propto$ and δ are implicated in the synthesis of the lagging and leading DNA strands respectively [Campbell, 1988, Leegwater *et al.*, 1991]. Despite their obvious importance, relatively little is known about DNA polymerases of parasitic protozoa. More research in this area will not only add to knowledge on the molecular biology of parasitic protozoa, but may lead to the development of more effective anti-parasite drugs. Here we describe our strategy for the cloning of a DNA polymerase gene of *T. gondii*.

NATO ASI Series, Vol. H 78
Toxoplasmosis
Edited by Judith E. Smith
© Springer-Verlag Berlin Heidelberg 1993

Results and Discussion

There are several possible strategies which can be used to clone genes encoding DNA polymerases. One involves immunoscreening expression libraries with an antiserum raised against the purified enzyme. The application of this approach to the isolation of DNA polymerase genes from *T. gondii* is difficult and limited principally by the large amount of parasite material needed for the purification. Another, and more commonly used approach, involves screening genomic or cDNA libraries with DNA probes. This approach has now been used successfully in isolating DNA polymerase genes from *Trypanosoma brucei* [Leegwater *et al.*, 1991] and *Plasmodium falciparum* [Ridley *et al.*, 1991]. In this respect, sequence analysis of DNA polymerase genes from a wide variety of organisms (including viruses, lower and higher eukaryotes) has shown that there are six conserved amino acid sequence regions (Figure 1; Wong *et al.*, 1988). In each case, the six regions are in the same spatial arrangement although the distances between them in the polypeptide of different organisms may vary. Thus, DNA sequences derived from these conserved regions may be useful as probes. Consequently, the cloned yeast DNA polymerase ∝ gene [Pizzagalli *et al.*, 1988] was obtained and two restriction fragments which covered the conserved regions I and II were isolated. However, neither of these two probes hybridised to *T. gondii* genomic DNA (data not shown).

$$\text{IV} \qquad \text{II VI III} \qquad \text{I} \quad \text{V}$$
$$\text{NH}_2 \text{ -----------O--------O--O--O-------O---O---------COOH}$$

Figure 1 Spatial arrangement of conserved sequences within a typical Pol ∝ polypeptide.

In parallel to the use of heterologous DNA probes, an approach involving the design and use of synthetic oligonucleotide probes was investigated. The DNA sequences of DNA polymerase genes from a variety of organisms are now known [Ito and Braithwaite, 1991]. Consequently, the DNA sequences of region II identified in genes of human [Wong *et al*, 1988], yeast [Pizzagalli *et al.*, 1988] and *T. brucei* [Leegwater *et al.*, 1991] were extracted and aligned (Figure 2). These organisms were chosen for analysis because they are eukaryotes whose genomic DNA base composition may be considered to be similar to that of *T. gondii*. They also represent a group of organisms which are not closely related. It is therefore likely that any conserved sequence identified among them may be present in the corresponding gene of *T. gondii*.

At 36 of the 57 base positions studied around Region II, identical bases were present in all three genes. A synthetic oligonucleotide probe was therefore designed on this region, and which included these conserved bases. The bases incorporated at the remaining 21 positions were chosen following compilation of a codon usage table, which was derived from eight genes of *T. gondii* that were located in Genbank (Accession Nos. J04018, M23658, M26007, M33472, M33572, M20024, M20025, M71274; Johnson, 1990; Ellis *et al.*, submitted). Southern hybridisation of this oligonucleotide probe to restriction digests of *T. gondii* established empirically the conditions necessary for hybridisation of this probe. Subsequently a *T. gondii* RH strain tachyzoite genomic DNA library (in lambda GEM-11) was screened using this oligonucleotide probe and two clones were identified by virtue of their positive hybridisation. The insert DNAs carried by them were analysed and found to be approximately 15 and 11 kb in size.

Since the *T. gondii* used to obtain parasite DNA were grown in the peritoneal cavities of mice, it is probable that the lambda GEM-11 library also contained murine genes. Although it is possible to isolate *T. gondii* DNA free of murine DNA [Johnson *et al.*, 1986], the separation is based on buoyant density centrifugation. Therefore not all of the parasite genomic DNA may be isolated, and hence this may not be ideal for producing *T. gondii* genomic libraries. Consequently, we chose to accept that our *T. gondii* library would contain murine genes, and decided to confirm that any clones giving a positive hybridisation signal with our oligonucleotide probe would have to be reanalysed to confirm that they were not of murine origin. Therefore the two cloned DNA's were hybridised to Southern blots containing *Eco R*1 digested murine and *T. gondii* DNA. The results obtained clearly showed that both cloned DNA's were derived from the *T. gondii* genome (Figure 3). Restriction enzyme (*Bam H*I, *Eco R*I, *Hind*III, *Sac* I) patterns of the two cloned gene inserts suggested that they were identical (data not shown).

Figure 2   Alignment of DNA sequences from region II of various DNA polymerase genes.

AMINO ACID	Asp	Phe	Asn	Ser	Leu	Tyr	Pro	Ser	Ile	Ile	Gln	Glu	Phe	Asn	Ile	Cys	Phe	Thr	Thr
HUMAN	GAC	TTC	AAC	AGT	CTA	TAT	CCT	TTC	ATC	ATT	CAG	GAA	TTT	AAC	ATT	TGT	TTT	ACA	ACA
YEAST	GAC	TTT	AAT	TCT	TTG	TAT	CCA	TCT	AAT	ATC	CAG	GAA	TTT	AAT	ATA	TGT	TTT	ACC	ACC
T. brucei	GAC	TTC	AAT	TCA	CTT	TGT	CCT	TCG	CTG	ATT	CAG	GAA	TTC	AAT	GTC	TGC	TAT	ACT	ACC
	* * *	* *	**	*	* *	*	**	**	*	**********	**	*	***	*	*				
T. gondii	GAC	TTC	AAT	TCT	CTC	TAT	CCC	TCT	ATC	ATT	CAG	GAA	TTC	AAC	ATT	TGC	TTC	ACC	ACC
		T			G	C	T C		C					G					

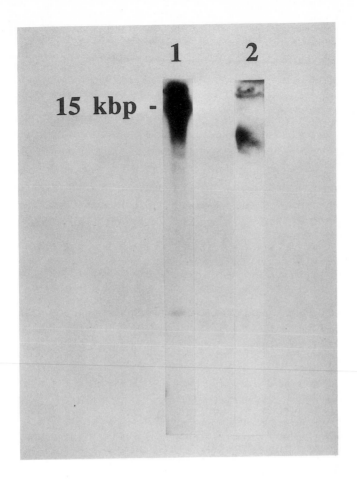

15 kbp -

Figure 3. Southern blots of (Lane 1 - *T. gondii*; Lane 2 - murine) DNA restricted with *Eco R*1 and hybridised with a radiolabelled purified clone from the *T. gondii* lambda GEM-11 library.

More than 40 different DNA polymerase enzymes have now been described [Ito and Braithwaite, 1991], although only limited information is available on these enzymes from parasite sources. Since DNA polymerases have been identified as possible targets for the rational design of antiparasitic drugs [Chang *et al.*, 1980; Solari *et al.*, 1983; de Vries *et al.*, 1991] more information is required about them. However the scarcity of parasite starting material has in general prevented the purification of polymerase enzymes which would assist in the study of their biochemistry. The cloning of DNA polymerase genes from different parasites has been seen to aid in the development of alternative methods of purification [Ridley *et al.*, 1991]. The genes encoding a DNA polymerase ∝ of *P. falciparum* and *T. brucei*, and a DNA polymerase δ of *P. falciparum* have been cloned by approaches similar to that described here using oligonucleotide probes homologous to a conserved region present in the gene sequence [Leegwater *et al.*, 1991; Ridley *et al.*, 1991]. The availability of the cloned gene from *T. gondii* will now assist, firstly in our studies on the replication of these organisms (and hence the development of vaccines), and secondly may allow the rational development of less toxic drugs which can be used to control infections of this organism in immunocompromised individuals.

REFERENCES

Campbell, J.L. (1986) Eukaryotic DNA replication. Ann. Rev. Biochem. 55 : 733-771.

Campbell, J.L. (1988) Eukaryotic DNA replication : yeast bares it ARS's. TIBS. 13 : 212-217.

Chang, L.M.S., Cheriathundam, E., Mahoney, E.M. and Cerami, A. (1980) DNA polymerases in parasitic protozoans differ from host enzymes. Science 208 : 510-511.

de Vries, E., Stam, J.G., Franssen, F.F.J., Nieuwenhuijs, H., Chavalitshewinkoon, P., de Clercq, E., Overdulve, J.P., and van der Vliet, P.C. (1991) Inhibition of the growth of *Plasmodium falciparum* and *Plasmodium berghei* by the DNA polymerase inhibitor HPMPA. Mol. Biochem. Parasitol. 47 : 43-50.

Ellis, J. and Johnson, A.M. (1992) Control of Intracellular Parasites: The Coccidia, in Control of Animal Parasites using Biotechnology, Yong, W.K. (Ed). CRC Press Inc., Boca Raton, In Press.

Ellis, J., Griffin, H., Morrison, D. and Johnson, A.M. (submitted). Dinucleotide frequency and codon usage in the phylum Apicomplexa.

Ito, J. and Braithwaite, D. (1991) Compilation and alignment of DNA polymerase sequences. Nucl. Acids. Res. 19 : 4045-4057.

Johnson, A.M., Dubey, J.P. and Dame, J.B. (1986) Purification and characterization of *Toxoplasma gondii* tachyzoite DNA. Aust. J. Exp. Biol. Med. Sci. 64 : 351-355.

Johnson, A.M. (1989) *Toxoplasma* Vaccines, in Veterinary Protozoan and Hemoparasite Vaccines, Wright, I.G. (Ed). CRC Press Inc., Boca Raton, p172.

Johnson, A.M. (1990) Comparison of dinucleotide frequency and codon usage in *Toxoplasma* and *Plasmodium* : evolutionary implications. J. Mol. Evol. 30 : 383-387.

Leegwater, P.A.J. Strating, M., Murphy, N.B., Kooy, R.F., van der Vliet, P.C. and Overdulve, J.P. (1991) The *Trypanosoma brucei* DNA polymerase $\propto$ core subunit gene is developmentally regulated and linked to constitutively expressed open reading frame. Nucl. Acids. Res. 19 : 6 41-6442.

McLeod, R., Mack, D. and Brown, C. (1991) *Toxoplasma gondii* : New advances in cellular and molecular biology. Exp. Parasitol. 72 : 109-121.

Ossorio, P.N., Schwartzman, J.D. and Boothroyd, J.C. (1992) A *Toxoplasma gondii* rhoptry protein associated with host cell penetration has unusual charge asymmetry. Mol. Biochem. Parasitol. 50 : 1-16.

Parmley, S.F., Sgarlato, G.D., Mark, J., Prince, J.B. and Remington, J.S. (1992). Expression, characterization and serologic reactivity of recombinant surface antigen P22 of *Toxoplasma gondii*. J. Clin. Micro. 30 : 1127-1133.

Pizzagalli, A., Valsasnini, P., Plevani, P. and Lucchini, G. (1988) DNA polymerase I gene of *Saccharomyces cerevisiae* : nucleotide sequence, mapping of a temperature-sensitive mutation, and protein homology with other DNA polymerases. Proc. Natl. Acad. Sci. USA 85 : 3772-3776.

Ridley, R.G., White, J.H., McAleese, S.M., Goman, M., Alano, P., de Vries, E. and Kilbey, B.J. (1991) DNA polymerase δ : gene sequences from *Plasmodium falciparum* indicate that this enzyme is more highly conserved that DNA polymerase $\propto$. Nucl. Acids. Res. 19 : 6731-6736.

Solari, A., Tharaud, Y, Repetto, J., Aldunate, J., Morello, A., an(1983) *In vitro* and *in vivo* studies of *Trypanosoma cruzi* DNA polymerase. Biochem. Int. 7 : 147-157.

Wang, T.S.F. (1991) Eukaryotic DNA polymerases. Ann. Rev. Biochem. 60 : 513-552.

Wong, S.W., Wah, A.F., Yuan, P-M., Arai, N., Perason, B.E., Arai, K., Korn, D., Hunkapiller, M.W. Wang, T.S.F. (1988) Human DNA polymerase ∝ gene expression is cell proliferation dependent and its primary structure is similar to both prokaryotic and eukaryotic replicative DNA polymerases. EMBO J. 7 : 37-47.

EXTRACHROMOSOMAL DNA IN THE APICOMPLEXA

Iain Wilson, Malcolm Gardner[*], Kaveri Rangachari, and
Don Williamson.
National Institute for Medical Research
Mill Hill
London NW7 1AA
U.K.

Extrachromosomal DNA adds a new dimension to genetic studies in the Apicomplexa. At a fundamental level, it has the potential to give a new perspective on evolutionary relationships between various taxa. Unlike the polymorphic diversity of many malarial chromosomal genes, a high level of sequence conservation is apparent in the malarial extrachromosomal DNAs that have been examined [Feagin, 1992] suggesting that they will be useful in tracing the evolution of taxa and genetically defined populations. In addition, and in more practical terms, analysis of extrachromosomal DNA may help with the application of specific chemotherapeutic intervention to organellar metabolic pathways. Although it might be argued that these aspects are rather limited, the finding that in malaria there are two unrelated forms of extrachromosomal DNA with organellar characteristics [Wilson et al., 1991; Feagin et al., 1992] is both unexpected and of general scientific interest. Consequently, a full description of the extrachromosomal DNAs in Apicomplexans should be made to complement other studies, such as the construction of chromosomal maps, that aim to improve our understanding of the genetics of important pathogenic organisms like *Toxoplasma* and *Plasmodium*.

----

*   Division of Experimental Therapeutics, Walter Reed Army
       Institute of Research, Washington, D.C. 20307-5100, U.S.A.

NATO ASI Series, Vol. H 78
Toxoplasmosis
Edited by Judith E. Smith
© Springer-Verlag Berlin Heidelberg 1993

Studies on extrachromosomal DNA in *Toxoplasma gondii* began in 1984 with the description of a circular DNA molecule, 11.6 μm in length [Borst et al., 1984]. This molecule formed a striking cruciform structure with arms 0.5 μm long and from denaturation/renaturation experiments it was inferred that the cruciform was part of an inverted repeat, circa 1.7 μm long, the length of the cruciform arms being determined by torsional restraints on the rest of the molecule. Drawing on knowledge of other extrachromosomal DNAs, Borst and his colleagues proposed that the circular DNA was the mitochondrial genome of *T.gondii* and inferred that the inverted repeat encoded rRNAs.

At about the same time, we isolated a similar circular DNA molecule with cruciform arms of 0.5 μm, from the simian malaria parasite *Plasmodium knowlesi* [Williamson et al., 1985]. What appeared to be replicating "theta-forms" were seen in some DNA preparations. This purified circular DNA was used as a probe to detect an homologous circular molecule in *P.falciparum*, of which we have cloned and sequenced about two thirds in the intervening years. The results of this work strongly suggest that the circular molecule is not mitochondrial DNA as was originally thought. We have proposed instead that it is the residual plastid genome of an ancient photosynthetic progenitor of this group of organisms [Wilson et al., 1991]. Evidence from other quarters suggests that the mitochondrial genome is encoded by a separate linear element, at least in malaria [Vaidya et al., 1989; Joseph et al., 1989; Feagin, 1992], *Toxoplasma* [Joseph et al., 1989] and *Theileria* [Megson et al., 1991].

Our proposal that the circular DNA in malaria is a residual plastid genome is still based on circumstantial evidence, and several decisive molecular phylogenetic questions remain to be answered [reviewed Palmer, 1992]. Stated simply, the present lines of evidence are the following: 1) only two forms of organellar extrachromosomal DNA are known in eukaryotes - mitochondrial (mt) and plastid (pt), and only one of the malarial extrachromosmal DNAs, the 6kb element, has mt characteristics; 2) a striking feature of ptDNAs is an inverted repeat containing rRNA genes [Palmer, 1985] - this is a dominant feature of the malarial circular DNA (Fig.1) although the organization of the inverted repeat is different from that of any known ptDNA; 3) unlike mtDNA, a characteristic of ptDNA is that it encodes genes for subunits of a eubacterial-like RNA polymerase - the presence of an *rpo*B/C operon on the malarial circular DNA is striking, indeed, the organization of the malarial *rpo*B gene is more like that of plastids than eubacteria (Gardner et al., 1991 and unpublished). Phylogenetic comparisons with the small number of *rpo*B/C sequences available in the database have shown that, whilst the malarial genes are distantly related to the others, the most closely related sequences available are those of *Euglena* ptDNA [Howe, 1992; and Gardner et al., unpublished]; 4) non-photosynthetic plants such as *Epiphagus virginiana* have residual pt genomes that characteristically retain genes involved in transcription and translation (rRNAs, tRNAs, ribosomal proteins, RNA polymerase subunits) [Morden et al., 1991] similar to those we have described on the malarial circle. Consequently, we have proposed, on the basis of its genetic content, that the malarial circular DNA resembles the residual ptDNA of achlorophyllous plants.

If the phylum Apicomplexa is monophyletic, currently a topic of debate [Johnson et al., 1987,1988; Barta et al., 1991; Gajadhar et al., 1991], it follows that homologues of both extrachromosomal DNAs are likely to be present in all members of the phylum. Evidence to substantiate this view is presented here with special reference to *Toxoplasma*.

ptDNA

What evidence is there that other Apicomplexan parasites contain a homologue of the ptDNA of malaria parasites? As mentioned above, a circular molecule with similar physical characteristics has been isolated from *Toxoplasma gondii*. More definitively, we have taken cloned DNA corresponding to portions of the small subunit (SSU) rRNA, large subunit (LSU) rRNA, and the *rpo*B genes of the *P.falciparum* circle and hybridized them to Southern blots of both endonuclease-restricted and unrestricted DNA from *T.gondii* and *Eimeria tenella*. All of the probes hybridized to the heterologous DNAs, giving bands of similar size to those found with the *P.falciparum* circle itself (Gardner et al., in preparation and Fig.2). Moreover, we exploited a characteristic feature of the malarial circle, namely its inverted repeat, to demonstrate that the cruciform structure in both *T.gondii* and *P.falciparum* circular DNAs is derived from the uniquely organized rRNA genes shown in Fig.1. Using restriction digests, complementary strands of duplicated sequences in the inverted repeat were allowed to snap-back following denaturation and renaturation, giving rise to hairpin molecules of greatly enhanced electrophoretic mobility. That the altered mobility is due to snap-back within the inverted repeat was demonstrated by selecting endonuclease restriction sites within and between the sequenced LSU and SSU rRNAs to generate a series of fragments of predictable size. All of these fragments were converted into rapidly migrating forms following denaturation and snap-back. In addition, when the undenatured and renatured

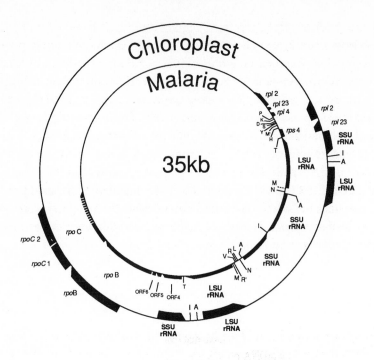

Figure 1. Comparison of the genetic organization of the malarial 35 kb circle with corresponding genes on chloroplast DNA; inner circle (*P.falciparum*) outer circle (*Marchantia polymorpha*). Genes for small and large subunit ribosomal RNAs (SSU and LSU rRNA), ribosomal proteins (*rps* and *rpl*), RNA polymerase subunits (*rpo*B/C), unidentified open reading frames (ORFs), and tRNAs (single letter amino acid code) are shown.

aliquots of the HpaI digest shown in Fig.2 were electrophoresed on an alkaline denaturing gel, each gave a single band of a size consistent with single strands of the native HpaI fragment. With *Plasmodium, Toxoplasma* and *Eimeria* there also was evidence that a proportion of the DNA spontaneously adopted the rapidly migrating form without the intervention of denaturation (Fig.2 lanes a). Although these results point to a high degree of conservation of the circular DNA, there is sequence diversity, even within different species of *Plasmodium*, that affects the symmetry of the restriction sites, obviating their use in snap-back experiments - see *P.chabaudi* in Fig.2. In short, the dimensions of the inverted repeat deduced by Borst and his colleagues for *T.gondii* correspond exactly to those we have found in the sequenced inverted repeat of *P. falciparum*, namely ~5100 nucleotides, equivalent to 1.7 µm (Fig.1). The span of the palindrome is thus 3.4 µm, approximately one third of the circle.

mtDNA

Comparative studies of mtDNA in the Apicomplexa are still rudimentary. Extracellular forms of *Toxoplasma* have a single large, branched, tubular mitochondrion that can be visualized with the fluorescent cationic dye rhodamine 123, as in *Plasmodium* [Divo et al., 1985]. Unlike *P. falciparum*, however, the *Toxoplasma* mitochondrion has well defined cristae. Vital staining of the mitochondrion did not occur when *T.gondii* was intracellular and it was proposed that the membrane potential might be reduced following inactivation of the mitochondrial electron transport system; however, other explanations remain possible [Tanabe & Murakami, 1984].

An extrachromosomal DNA corresponding to the 6kb element of malaria parasites was identified in *T.gondii* following caesium chloride density gradient separation of total DNA and cross-hybridization with a malarial probe [Joseph et al., 1989]. In *Plasmodium* the 6kb element encodes fragmented rRNA genes and three open reading frames homologous to the mitochondrial protein coding genes cytochrome oxidase, subunits I and III, and cytochrome b [Feagin, 1992]. In *T.gondii*, fragments of the mitochondrial genes cytochrome oxidase subunit 1 (*cox*I) and cytochrome b (*cyt*b), bounded by a 91 base pair repeat, have been found integrated into chromosomal DNA [Ossorio et al., 1991]. It is presumed that *Toxoplasma* mitochondria have a direct analogue of the 6kb element of *Plasmodium* but this has still to be characterized.

A difference between *Toxoplasma, Eimeria* and *Plasmodium* that might have

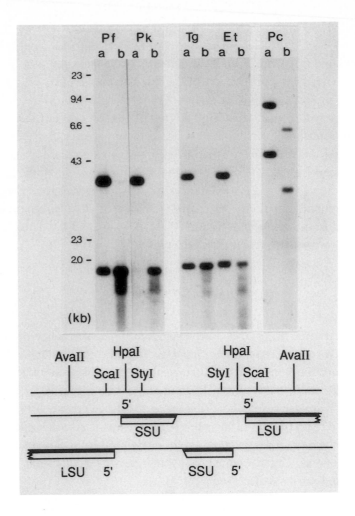

Figure 2. Top. Southern blot of *Hpa*I digested parasite DNAs, without (a) and with (b) snapback treatment. The restriction fragments were hybridized to a probe for Pf 35 kb small subunit rRNA. Pf, *Plasmodium falciparum;* Pk, *Plasmodium knowlesi;* Pc, *Plasmodium chabaudi;* Tg, *Toxoplasma gondii;* Et, *Eimeria tenella.* Fragment sizes are indicated (kb). Bottom. Restriction sites used for snapback experiments.

important implications for studies on the inheritance of mtDNA and the generation of diversity is that, on the basis of morphological evidence, the microgametes of *Toxoplasma* and *Eimeria* have a mitochondrion [Scholtysech et al., 1972] whereas *Plasmodium* does not [Aikawa et al., 1984]. In agreement with this last conclusion, we have found that inheritance of the *cyt*b gene in *P.falciparum* is uniparental [Creasey et al., in preparation]. This was established from the inheritance pattern of a single nucleotide difference in the *cyt*b gene of two cloned lines of *P.falciparum* which were crossed. Because it is not possible at present to separate viable male and female gametes, we are not able to say definitively which gamete carried the mtDNA into the zygote. However, on the basis of the electron microscopic evidence cited above, only the macrogamete is believed to contain a mitochondrion. The development of extrachromosmal markers which are inherited in a uniparental fashion, without the opportunity for recombination evident in many nuclear genes, should be useful in tracing the evolution of populations of *Plasmodium*. The fate of the microgamete's mitochondrion at zygote formation in *Toxoplasma* remains to be determined.

Another interesting difference amongst Apicomplexans is that mtDNA appears to be in different physical forms. For example, *Theileria* and *Babesia* have a linear element of about 7kb although the genetic content is similar to the 6kb tandemly repeated element of *Plasmodium* [Nene et al., 1992]. The linear molecule is believed to have ends protected by tandem repeats reminiscent of, but different from, the telomeres on the mtDNA of *Tetrahymena thermophila* [Morin and Cech, 1986]. This form of mtDNA must be maintained by a different mode of replication from the tandemly repeated element in *Plasmodium* which may be generated by a rolling circle mechanism [Preiser & Williamson, unpublished]. Clearly, there is still a great deal to learn about the mtDNAs of the Apicomplexa before an overall picture can be discerned.

Acknowledgement.

This investigation received financial support from the UNDP/World Bank/WHO Special Programme for Research and Training in Tropical Diseases (TDR).

References

Aikawa, M., Carter, R., Ito, Y., Nijhout, M.N. [1984] New observations on gametogenesis, fertilization, and zygote formation in *Plasmodium falciparum*. J. Protozool 31: 403-413.

Barta, J.R., Jenkins, M.C., Danforth, H.D., [1991] Evolutionary relationships avaian *Eimeria* species among other Apicomplexan protozoa: Monophyly of the Apicomplexa is supported. Mol Biol Evol 8: 345-355.

Borst, P., Overdulve, J.P., Weijers, P.J., Fase-Fowler, F., Van Den Berg, M. [1984] DNA circles with cruciforms from *Isospora (Toxoplasma) gondii*. Biochem Biophys Acta 781: 100-111.

Creasey, A., Ranford-Cartwright, L.C., Balfe, P., Walliker, D., Moore, D., Williamson, D.H., Wilson, R.J.M., Carter, R. [1992] Uniparental inheritance of the cytochrome b gene in *Plasmodium falciparum*. In preparation.

Divo, A.A., Geary, T.G., Jensen, J.B., Ginsburg, H. [1985] The mitochondrion of *Plasmodium falciparum* visualized by rhodamine 123 fluorescence. J. Protozool 32: 442-446.

Feagin, J.E., [1992] The 6kb element of *Plasmodium falciparum* encodes mitochondrial cytochrome genes. Mol Biochem parasitol 52: 145-148.

Feagin, J.E., Werner, E., Garner, M.J., Williamson, D.H., Wilson R.J.M. [1992] Homologies between the contiguous and fragmented rRNAS of the two *Plasmodium falciparum* extrachromosomal DNAs are limited to core sequences. Nuc Acids Res 20: 879-887.

Gajadhar, A.A., Marquardt, W.C., Hall, R., Gunderson, J., Aritzia Carmona, E.V., Sogin, M.L. [1991] Ribosomal RNA sequences of *Sarcocystis muris*, *Theileria annulata* and *Crypthecodinium cohnii* reveal evolutionary relationships among apicomplexans, dinoflagellates, and ciliates. Mol Biochem Parasitol 45: 147-154.

Gardner, M.J., Williamson, D.H., Wilson, R.J.M. [1991] A circular DNA in malaria parasites encodes an RNA polymerase like that of prokaryotes and chloroplasts. Mol Biochem Parasitol 44: 115-124.

Howe, C. [1992] Plastid origin of an extrachromosomal DNA molecule from *Plasmodium*, causative agent of malaria. J Theor Biol. In press.

Johnson, A.M., Murray, P.J., Illana, S., Baverstock, P.J. [1987] Rapid nucleotide sequence analysis of the small subunit ribosomal RNA of *Toxoplasma gondii*: evolutinary implications for the Apicomplexa. Mol Biochem Parasitol 25: 239-246.

Joseph, J.T., Aldritt, S.M., Unnasch, T., Puijalon, U., Wirth, D. [1989] Characterization of a conserved extrachromosomal element isolated from the avian malarial parasite *Plasmodium gallinaceum*. Mol Cell Biol 9: 3621-3629.

Megson, A., Inman, G.J., Hunt, P.D., Baylis, H.A., Hall, R. [1991] The gene for apocytochrome B of *Theileria annulata* resides on a small linear extrachromosomal element. Mol Biochem Parasitol 48: 113-116.

Morden, C.W., Wolfe, K.H., dePamphilis, C.W., Palmer, J.D. [1991] Plastid translation and transcription genes in a non-photosynthetic plant: intact, missing and pseudo genes. EMBO J 10: 3281-3288.

Morin, G.B., Cech, T.R. [1986] The telomeres of the linear mitochondrial DNA of *Tetrahymena thermophila* consist of 53 bp tandem repeats. Cell: 10: 873-883.

Nene, V., Gobright, E., Kairo, A [1992] A subset of *Theileria parva* mitochondrial proteins is encoded by a linear 7.1 kbp DNA molecule. J Cell Bio Suppl 16a: 116.

Ossorio, P.N., Sibley, L.D., Boothroyd, J.C. [1991] Mitochondrial-like DNA sequences flanked by direct and inverted repeats in the nuclear genome of *Toxoplasma gondii*. J. Mol Biol 222: 525-536.

Palmer, J.D., [1985] Comparative organization of chloroplast genomes. Ann Rev Genet 19: 325-354.

Palmer, J.D. [1992] Green ancestry of malarial parasites? Curr Biol 2: 318-320.

Scholtysech, E., Mehlhorn, H., Hammond, D.M., [1972] Electron microscopic studies of microgametogenesis in coccidia and related groups. Z Parasitenk 38: 95-131.

Tanabe, K., Murakami, K [1984] Reduction in the mitochondrial membrane potential of *Toxoplasma gondii* after invasion of host cells. J Cell Sci 70: 73-81.

Vaidya, A.B., Akella, R., Suplick, K. [1989] Sequences similar to two mitochondrial proteins and portions of ribosomal RNA in tandemly arrayed 6-kilobase-pair DNA of a malarial parasite. Mol Biochem Parasitol 35: 97-108 and Corrigendum 39: 295-296.

Williamson, D.H., Wilson, R.J.M., Bates, P.A., McCready, S., Perler, F., Qiang, B [1985]. Nuclear and mitochondrial DNA of the primate malarial parasite *Plasmodium knowlesi*. Mol Biochem Parasitol 14: 199-209.

Wilson, R.J.M., Gardner, M.J., Feagin, J.E., Williamson, D.H., [1991] Have malaria parasites three genomes? Parasitology Today 7: 134-136.

CELL BIOLOGY
OF
TOXOPLASMA

FORMATION AND MODIFICATION OF THE PARASITOPHOROUS VACUOLE OCCUPIED BY *TOXOPLASMA GONDII*

L. David Sibley, Christine Pouletty, and John C. Boothroyd
Department of Molecular Microbiology
Washington University School of Medicine
St. Louis, MO 63110 USA

Introduction

Toxoplasma tachyzoites are able to actively invade and survive within specialized vacuoles in a wide range of vertebrate host cells. The parasite enters a vacuole that is derived from the plasma membrane by invagination, yet these vacuoles differ from standard phagocytic compartments in several respects. The Toxoplasma-containing vacuole, or parasitophorous vacuole (PV), resists acidification [Sibley et al., 1985b] and fusion with lysosomes [Jones and Hirsch 1972]. These vacuoles also resist fusion with vesicles containing soluble tracers for fluid phase endocytosis including Lucifer yellow [Joiner et al., 1990] and with vesicles containing permanent labels such as acridine orange that accumulate in acidic compartments [Sibley et al., 1985a]. While the PV is inert with respect to interactions with the host-cell endocytic network, events within the vacuole are dynamic. During invasion and vacuole formation, the parasite secretes a number of proteins from specialized storage organelles called rhoptries and dense granules. The contents of these secretory organelles are targetted to different sites within the vacuole including the vacuolar membrane and the intravacuolar network that forms a membranous interface within the vacuole [Sibley et al., 1986].

Our initial purification of this intravacuolar network demonstrated that it is comprised of secretory proteins stored within cytoplasmic vesicles in the parasite that are released following invasion [Sibley and Krahenbuhl 1988; Sibley 1989]. More recently, it has been shown that the dense granules are the storage site for a number of these secretory proteins including : GRA1, a 23kD calcium binding protein [Cesbron-Delauw et al., 1989], GRA2 (p28),

---

Department of Microbiology and Immunology, Standford University, School of Medicine, Standford, CA, 94305, USA.

NATO ASI Series, Vol. H 78
Toxoplasmosis
Edited by Judith E. Smith
© Springer-Verlag Berlin Heidelberg 1993

Table 1.   Endogenous markers for the host cell endocytic pathway.

COMPARTMENT	MARKER	ANTIBODY	
Plasma Membrane	TfR	R-Pc	[1]
	ManR	R-Pc	[2]
Coated Pits	CLATHRIN	X22	[3]
	ADAPTIN-2	AP.6	[3]
Early Endomsome	TfR	R-Pc	[1]
	ENDOLYN	2C5	[4]
Late Endosome	MPR	R-Pc	[5]
	ENDOLYN	2C5	[4]
	LAMPs	1D4B	[6]
		ABL93	[6]
Trans Golgi Network	CLATHRIN	X-22	[3]
	MPR	R-Pc	[5]
Lysosomes	ENDOLYN	2C5	[4]
	LAMPs	1D4B	[6]
		ABL93	[6]

Pc refers to polyclonal antisera, monoclonals are referred to by name. TfR, Transferrin receptor, ManR, Mannose/fucose receptor, MPR, cation-independent mannose-6 phosphate receptor, LAMPs, lysosome associated membrane proteins. [1] H. Sussman, Stanford University, [2] P. Stahl, Washington University, [3] F. Brodsky, UCSF, [4] M. Rosenfeld, NYU, [5] S. Pfeffer, Stanford University, [6] T. August, John Hopkins University.

We have previously reported that the pH of the *Toxoplasma* PV remains near neutral after formation in normal macrophages and postulated that the resistance of *Toxoplasma* PVs to acidification must proceed either by active inhibition or by exclusion of host components from the vacuole [Sibley et al., 1985b]. To examine the mechanism by which the PV avoids acidification, we have used newly characterized monoclonal antibodies to the proton pump found in endosomes and lysosomes (antibodies obtained from Dr Steve Gluck, Washington University [Yurko and Gluck 1987]). Newly formed *Toxoplasma* PVs in MDBK and NRK cells do not contain detectable amounts of the proton pump as verified by immunofluorescence microscopy. Similarly, in bone marrow-derived mouse macrophages, the proton pump is excluded from newly formed *Toxoplasma* PVs. In part, this result can be attributed to the avoidance of fusion with other endocytic compartments as discussed above.

However, the complete absence of markers for early endosomes and of the proton pump, suggests that these components are actively excluded from the vacuole at the time of formation. This novel ability may be related to an unique mechanism of cell entry that excludes intramembranous particles during formation of the vacuole through a moving junction at the parasite-host interface [Porchet-Hennere and Torpier 1983].

When *Toxoplasma* cells are first coated with specific antibodies, they enter vacuoles in macrophages that rapidly become positive for the proton pump. These compartments also rapidly acquire other markers of endocytic processing including mannose/fucose receptors and LAMPs. This result is consistent with previous observations that antibody opsonized *Toxoplasma* enter vacuoles that undergo very rapid acidification [Sibley et al., 1985b], and ultimately fuse with lysosomes [Jones and Hirsch 1972]. Importantly, Fc receptor-mediated opsonization is also capable of targeting *Toxoplasma* to lysosomes in non-phagocytic CHO cells [Joiner et al., 1990].

The nonfusigenic nature of the *Toxoplasma* PV may be related to the rapid modification of this compartment by secretion of parasite proteins and/or lipids during invasion. In addition to rhoptry and dense granule components, parasite surface proteins are shed during and following invasion. The surface membrane protein p30 is partially shed during invasion and is often found as membrane blebs either at the host cell surface or in cytoplasmic vesicles separate from the PV [Dubremetz et al., 1985]. Intracellular tachyzoites retain much of their surface p30, indicating this process does not completely remove the surface protein coat.

In addition, we have observed that p30 can be readily visualized as a component of the vacuolar membrane, in clusters within the vacuole, in extensions of the PV, and in vesicles within the host cell cytoplasm that are separate from the PV. These structures form during the intracellular division of tachyzoites and are distinct from those described, during invasion, above. Detection of these forms of secreted p30 is dependent on the extraction procedures used to permeabilize cells after fixation and prior to immuno-labelling. As shown in figure 1, when Triton X-100 is used to extract cells, p30 is only seen associated with the plasma membrane of the tachyzoites. However, when saponin is used as a permeabilizing agent, p30 is clearly seen in the vacuolar membrane as well as the parasite plasma membrane. This

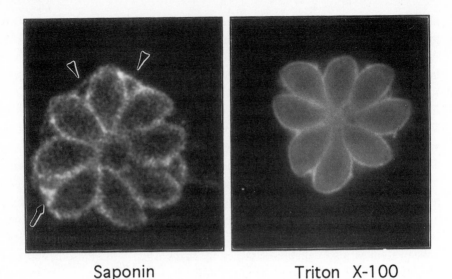

Saponin   Triton X-100

Figure 1. Immunofluorescence localization of p30 in infected human fibroblast cells. Extraction with saponin (left panel) retains p30 present in the vacuole membrane (arrowheads) and as clusters within the vacuole (arrow). In contrast, these forms of p30 are extracted when the cells are permeabilized with Triton X-100 (right panel). Immunostaining with mAb DG52 and FITC conjugated goat anti-mouse IgG.

difference may be related to the lipid anchor of p30 [Nagel and Boothroyd 1989] that renders it susceptible to extraction with Triton X-100 when it is found in the vacuolar membrane or intravacuolar network. The intracellular fate of these p30-containing vesicles, which are separate from the PV, may have significance to the pathways for antigen presentation in infected cells. We have previously reported that one of the major components of the intravacuolar network is a 32 kD protein that is secreted from dense granules

[Sibley and Krahenbuhl 1988]. These findings were obtained with the monoclonal antibody 1G5 (kindly provided by Dr Jack Remington). It was subsequently shown that 1G5 reacts strongly to reduced p30 both when purified from *Toxoplasma* cells and when expressed as a recombinant fusion protein in *E. coli* [Burg et al., 1988]. Further examination revealed that 1G5 reacts to an epitope on p30 that is partially shared by one or more independent gene products. The results that support this conclusion are briefly summarized as follows. First, 1G5 reacts to dense granules in tachyzoites when examined by immunofluorescence (confirming our earlier EM results [Sibley and Krahenbuhl 1988]) and this reaction is still seen in a p30 mutant that does not express any detectable form of the p30 protein [Kasper et al., 1992]. However, using a variety of other mAbs to p30, there is no indication that p30 is found in dense granules of wild type or p30-mutant tachyzoites. Second, 1G5 reacts weakly to several bands on non-reduced SDS PAGE blots that do not comigrate with native p30 but instead are similar in size to p28 (GRA2) and p29 (GRA3), both of which are exclusively located in dense granules.

To test the possibility that 1G5 cross reacts with a dense granule protein(s) we examined the reaction of 1G5 with recombinant p30 or with recombinant p28 (kindly provided by Dr Jack Remington) by SDS PAGE and immunoblotting. As seen in figure 2, 1G5 reacts strongly with reduced, recombinant p30. 1G5 also reacts with recombinant p28 with a significant, although less intense, staining than with its natural eptiope on p30. These results demonstrate that 1G5 reacts with an epitope on p30 that is partially shared by p28. In retrospect, it seems likely that our findings demonstrating the intravacuolar network forms by secretion of dense granule proteins into the PV were due in part to this fortuitous cross reaction. This does not invalidate the importance of dense granule secretion, as both our studies, discussed below, and numerous others have demonstrated the specific release of dense granules following invasion. Because of the cross reactive nature of 1G5, we have discontinued using this mAb for localization studies and have instead examined the secretion of dense granules using antibodies specific to recombinant p28.

The gene encoding p28 predicts an open reading frame of 252 amino acids with a single internal hydrophobic domain [Prince et al., 1989]. Using a rabbit polyclonal antiserum produced against recombinant p28 fused to ß-gal (kindly provided by Dr Jack Remington), we have examined the regulation of

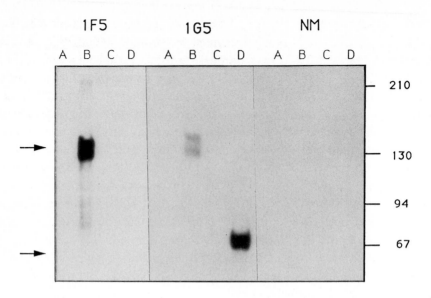

Figure 2. Western blot analysis of mAb 1G5 that reacts to p30 fusion protein and cross reacts to p28 fusion protein expressed in *E. coli*. For comparison the reaction of anti-p28 mAb, 1F5 (kindly provided by Jean Francois Dubremetz) is shown. Lanes refer to: A, β-gal vector control, B, β-gal fused tp p28 (contains amino acids 80 to 252 [Prince et al., 1989]; C, TrpE vector control, D, TrpE fused to full length p30 [Burg et al., 1988]. NM refers to normal mouse sera.

GRA2 secretion that follows invasion using confocal immunofluorescence and immunoEM localization.

Ultrastructurally, exocytosis of dense granules occurs by fusion of the granule membrane to the parasite plasma membrane and release of amorphous contents into the vacuole. A second type of dense granule secretion is observed at a specialized site that forms as an invagination of the posterior end [Sibley

1989]. Coincident with this posterior secretion, a large cluster of membranous tubules is released into the vacuole giving rise to the intravacuolar network described previously [Sibley et al., 1986]. This event is transitory and at later time points the posterior end returns to its normal convex, rounded shape. Ultrastructural evidence indicates this membranous network originates from a novel secretory granule that contains lipids and possible pre-formed membranes [Sibley 1989]. Components of the network fuse with the vacuolar membrane, connecting the tubular projections within the vacuole to the surrounding membrane in a continuous bilayer. This process of exocytosis of membrane constitutes a novel modification of the vacuolar membrane that may play a role in preventing fusion or in facilitating nutrient transport across this interface.

In extracellular tachyzoites, p28 is located within dense granules, visible as discrete dots of immunofluorescence. Following invasion, the dense granules coalesce and migrate to both poles of the cell. Secretion of dense granules occurs rapidly during the first 10 min after invasion and is detected at many places along the membrane where dense granules must first cross the inner membrane complex. Following release, p28 can be visualized as a cluster of immunofluorescence that lies adjacent to the parasite cell within the vacuole. ImmunoEM localization confirms that this distribution corresponds to the intravacuolar network. Several hours after infection, this cluster has dispersed and p28 is seen throughout the vacuole space in association with the tubular elements that make up the network. Although p28 is found at sites where the network makes direct contact with the vacuolar membrane, it does not transfer to the vacuole membrane, indicating a specific targeting process is involved. Although it has previously been published that p28 is also detected in the inner membrane complex or pellicle of the *Toxoplasma* cell [Charif et al., 1990] we have not observed this pattern of labelling with rabbit anti p-28 sera.

In previous studies we have shown that dense granule release is influenced by extracellular calcium levels [Sibley et al., 1986]. To further characterize the process of dense granule exocytosis, we have developed quantitative methods to examine the role of calcium in secretion by extracellular tachyzoites [Sibley and Boothroyd 1991]. The calcium ionophore A23187 stimulates p28 release from extracellular tachyzoites in a dose dependent manner. A23187-induced secretion is temperature dependent and not influenced by protonophores such as monensin. The kinetics of A23187 release by extracellular tachyzoites and the morphological appearance of granule fusion and exocytosis are similar to that observed during natural infection of host cells. Collectively these studies demonstrate an important role for calcium in regulating secretion of dense granules.

Acknowledgments

We are grateful to Jean-Francois Dubremetz, Steve Parmley, and Jack Remington for reagents and exchange of unpublished data.

References

Achbarou, A., Mercereau-Puijalon, O., Sadak, A., Fortier, B., Leriche, M.A., and Camus, D. [1991]. Differential targeting of dense granule proteins in the parasitophorous vacuole of *Toxoplasma gondii*. Parasitol. 103: 321-329.

Burg, J.L., Perlman, D., Kasper, L.H., Ware, P.L., and Boothroyd, J.C. [1988]. Molecular analysis of the gene encoding the major surface antigen of *Toxoplasma gondii*. J. Immunol. 141: 3584-3591.

Cesbron-Delauw, M.F., Guy, B. Pierce, R.J., Lenzen, G., Cesbron, J.Y. Charif, H., Lepage, P., Darcy, F., Lecocq, J.P., and Capron A., [1989]. Molecular characterization of a 23-kilodalton major antigen secreted by *Toxoplasma gondii*. Proc. Nat. Acad. Sci., USA 86: 7537-7541.

Charif, H., Darcy, F., Torpier, G., Cesbron-Delauw, M.F., and Capron, A. [1990]. *Toxoplasma gondii*: Characterization and localization of antigens secreted from tachyzoites. Exp. Parasitol. 71: 114-124.

Darcy, F., Deslee, D., Santoro, F., Charif, H., Auriault, C., Decoster, A., Duquesne, V. and Capron, A., [1988]. Induction of a protective anti-body dependent response against toxoplasmosis by *in vitro* excreted/secreted antigens from tachyzoites of *Toxoplasma gondii*. Paras. Immunol. 10: 553-567.

Decoster, A., Darcy, F., and Capron A. [1988]. Recognition of *Toxoplasma gondii* excreted and secreted antigens by human sera from acquired and congenital toxoplasmosis: Identification of markers of acute and chronic infection. Clin. Exp. Immunol. 73: 376-382.

Dubremetz, J.F., Rodriguez, C., and Ferreira E. [1985]. *Toxoplasma gondii*: Redistribution of monoclonal antibodies on tchyzoites during host cell invasion. Exp. Parasitol. 59: 24-32.

Joiner, K.A., Furhman, S.A., Miettinen, H.M., Kasper, L.H., and Mellman I. [1990]. Fusion competence of parasitophorous vacuoles in Fc receptor transfected fibroblasts. Science 249: 641-646.

Jones, T.C. and Hirsch J.G. [1972]. The interaction of *Toxoplasma gondii* and mammalian cells. II The absence of lysosomal fusion with phagocytic vacuoles containing living parasites. J. Exp. Med. 136: 1173-1194.

Kasper, L.H., Khan, I.A. Ely, K.H., Beulow R., and Boothroyd J.C. [1992]. Antigen-specific [p30] mouse CD8+ T cells are cytotoxic against *Toxoplasma gondii* - infected peritoneal macrophages. J. Immunol. 148: 1493-1498.

Leriche, M.A. and Dubremetz J.F. [1990]. Exocytosis of *Toxoplasma* dense granules into the parasitophorous vacuole after invasion. Parasitol. Res. 76: 359-362.

Leriche, M.A. and Dubremetz J.F., [1991]. Characterization of the protein contents of rhoptries and dense granule of *Toxoplasma gondii* tachyzoites by subcellular fractionation and monoclonal antibodies. Mol. Biochem. Parasitol. 45: 249-260.

Nagel, S.D. and Boothroyd, J.C. [1989]. The major surface antigen, p30, of *Toxoplasma gondii* is anchored by a glycolipid. J. Biochem. 264: 5569-5574.

Porchet-Hennere, E. and Torpier G. [1983]. Relations entre *Toxoplasma* et sa cellule-hote. Protistologica 19: 357-370.

Prince, J.B. Araujo, F.G., Remington, J.S., Burg, J.L., Boothroyd, J.C. and Sharma, S. [1989]. Cloning of cDNAs encoding a 28-kilodalton antigen of *Toxoplasma gondii*. Mol. Biochem. Parasitol. 34: 3-14.

Sibley, L.D. [1989]. Active modification of host cell phagosomes by *Toxoplasma gondii*. In: Intracellular Parasitism. Ed. J. Moulder, Boca Raton, CRC. 245-257.

Sibley, L.D. and Boothroyd J.C. [1991]. Calcium regulated secretion and modification of host-cell endocytic compartments by *Toxoplasma*. J. Cell Biol. 115: 5a.

Sibley, L.D. and Krahenbuhl J.L. [1988]. Modification of host cell phagosomes by *Toxoplasma gondii* involves redistribution of surface proteins and secretion of a 32 kDa protein. E.J. Cell Biol. 47: 81-87.

Sibley, L.D., Krahenbuhl, J.L., Adams, G.M.W., and Weidner, E., [1986]. *Toxoplasma* modifies macrophage phagosomes by secretion of a vesicular network rich in surface proteins. J. Cell Biol. 103: 867-874.

Sibley, L.D., Krahenbuhl, J.L., and Weidner, E., [1985a]. Lymphokine activation of J774G8 cells and mouse peritoneal macrophages challenged with *Toxoplasma gondii*. Infect. Immun. 49: 760-764.

Sibley, L.D., Weidner E., and Krahenbuhl, J.L. [1985b]. Phagosome acidification blocked by intracellular *Toxoplasma gondii*. Nature (Lond.) 315: 416-419.

Yurko, M.A. and Gluck, S. (1987). Production and characterization of a monoclonal antibody to vacuolar H+ATPase of renal epithelia. J. Biochem. 32: 15770-15779.

THE PARASITOPHOROUS VACUOLE MEMBRANE SURROUNDING *T. GONDII*: A SPECIALIZED INTERFACE BETWEEN PARASITE AND CELL

Keith A. Joiner
Section of Infectious Diseases
Department of Medicine
Yale University School of Medicine
New Haven, Connecticut
USA 06510-8056

Introduction

Cell invasion by apicomplexan parasites is a rapid yet highly ordered process dependent upon oriented attachment of the parasite to the target cell, parasite motility, and secretion of anterior organelles (rhoptries) during the invasion event (reviewed in Werk 1985). Subsequent to invasion of the host cell, the apicomplexan parasite, *Toxoplasma gondii*, resides within a specialized parasitophorous vacuole (PV). Unlike phagolysosomes, the parasitophorous vacuole neither fuses with lysosomes nor acidifies [Joiner et al. 1990; Jones and Hirsch 1972; Sibley et al. 1985].

Immediately following parasite entry into the host cell, the parasitophorous vacuole membrane (PVM) lacks observable transmembrane proteins [Porchet-Hennere and Torpier 1983], and appears by freeze fracture electron microscopy to be a phospholipid bilayer. Although this would be likely to contribute to the fusion incompetence of the vacuole [Joiner et al. 1990], such a membrane would impede access of the parasite to nutrients from the host cell.

As the vacuole matures, intramembranous particles, presumably representative of transmembrane proteins, appear progressively in the PVM [Porchet-Hennere and Torpier 1983; Dubremetz, unpublished observations]. We, and others, have hypothesized that these modifications of the vacuolar membrane are necessary for parasite survival. To explore this hypothesis, we are examining the composition of the vacuolar membrane immediately after its formation, the progressive modifications in the PVM which occur with time, and the consequences of these modifications on membrane transport of ions, nucleosides and antimicrobial agents. The underlying premise behind the experiments is that the vacuolar membrane is unique, is extensively modified

NATO ASI Series, Vol. H 78
Toxoplasmosis
Edited by Judith E. Smith
© Springer-Verlag Berlin Heidelberg 1993

by parasite components, and may represent either a therapeutic target or a drug delivery system.

A brief summary of our work on *T. gondii* is provided below, with emphasis on the ongoing projects and current directions of the laboratory.

Cell Attachment and Entry by *T. gondii*

In a series of recently completed papers, we have shown that laminin on the parasite surface mediates binding of tachyzoites to laminin receptors on host cells, receptors which differ depending upon the host cell type [Furtado et al. 1992a; Furtado et al. 1992b; Furtado et al. 1992c]. Although interesting, we do not currently plan to pursue these experiments further, allowing us to focus our efforts on the membrane transport events within the infected cell.

In a paper published several years ago [Joiner et al. 1990], we showed that the fusion competence of the vacuole containing *T. gondii* was dictated by the route of entry. Parasites which actively invaded Chinese Hamster Ovary fibroblasts formed vacuoles which were irreversibly fusion imcompetent, and did not fuse with any membrane-bound organelle of the host cell. In contrast, vacuoles containing antibody-coated parasites phagocytosed by CHO cells stably transfected with the murine low affinity FcRII receptor fused with endosomes and lysosomes and became acidified. We have extended these observations by doing analogous experiments with the human high affinity FcRI receptor [Cohen, Mellman, and Joiner, unpublished observations].

Modification of the Parasitophorous Vacuole Membrane Following Cell Entry

a)   Dense Granule Protein Secretion and Localization

Secretion of dense granule proteins into the vacuolar space is detected within 10 minutes after cell invasion, and continues progressively as the vacuole matures [Dubremetz, Ossorio and Joiner, in preparation]. Four dense granule proteins (GRA1, 2, 3 and 4) are idenified by monoclonal antibodies [Leriche and Dubremetz 1991]. GRA1, a 23 kDa calcium-binding protein, GRA2, a 28 kDa protein, and GRA4, a 40 kDa molecule, localize to a reticular network within the parasitophorous vacuole space [Cesbron-Delauw et al. 1989; Charif et al. 1990; Sibley and Krahenbuhl 1988; Sibley et al. 1986; Cesbron, this volume; Dubremetz, this volume; Sibley, this volume]. In contrast, of the currently characterized dense granule proteins, GRA 3 is unique in associating almost exclusively with the PVM [Achbarou et al. 1991; Dubremetz and Joiner, in preparation].

GRA3 associated with the parasitophorous vacuole membrane has a variety of different characteristics in comparison to GRA3 from extracellular tachyzoites [Ossorio, Dubremetz and Joiner, in preparation]. A portion of GRA3 from infected cells is present in a membrane frraction on sucrose flotation gradients, whereas GRA3 liberated from parasites remains at the loading interface. GRA3 associated with the PVM from infected cells partitions partially into the detergent phase of a TX114 partitioning scheme and is not released from the PVM by washing with 1M NaCl or Na_2CO_3. GRA 3 released from extracellular parasites partitions into the aqueous phase of a TX114 partitioning system and remains in a 100,000 x g supernatant. Hence, GRA 3 associated with the PVM has either undergone a conformational change associated with exposure of hydrophobic domains or has associated tightly with a hydrophobic membrane-associated molecule or complex. Experiments are underway to distinguish between these two possibilities.

b)   The Deduced Protein Sequence of GRA3 Includes a Putative Transmembrane Domain

A partial nucleotide sequence has been obtained for GRA3 [Bermudes, Dubremetz and Joiner, unpublished results]. Positive clones were identified by antibody screening (polyclonal and monoclonal) of a lambda gt11 cDNA library, kindly provided by Dr John Boothroyd. Antibodies affinity purified on the recombinant fusion protein recognize a 30 kDa protein by immunoblot and stain the PVM of infected cells. The deduced protein sequence is notable for the presence of a putative transmembrane domain. No significant homology with other proteins in the data base was noted.

c)   Parasite Proteins on the Cytoplasmic Face of the PVM

The orientation of GRA3 and additional parasite proteins within the PVM was investigated. The plasma membrane of cells infected with *T. gondii* was permeabilized with the pore forming bacterial toxin Streptolysin O or with the detergent digitonin under conditions in which the PVM was not permeabilized. This system allows access of antibody molecules to the cytoplasmic side of the PVM. Under these conditions, bright staining of the PVM was observed with antisera to whole *T. gondii* or with antisera to a rhoptry-dense granule preparation [Beckers, Dubremetz, and Joiner, unpublished observations].

GRA 3, however, was not readily detected by immunofluorescence on the cytoplasmic face of the PVM. It is possible that GRA3 epitopes on the cytoplasmic face of the PVM are not recognized by the available anti-GRA3 antibodies. Alternatively, the additional parasite proteins which are cytoplasmically disposed in the PVM [Beckers, Dubremetz and Joiner, unpublished observations] may be the major parasite components inserted into or transported through the PVM. Identification and characterization of these additional proteins is underway in our laboratory.

d)   The Parasitophorous Vacuole Membrane Contains a Putative Pore

The presence of a putative pore within the PVM has been demonstrated by microinjection of variously sized fluorescent tracers into the vacuolar space. Rapid flux of small molecules across the PVM has been shown [Schwab, Beckers and Joiner, in preparation].

Nucleoside Salvage by *T. gondii*

T. gondii, like all intracellular protozoa, is a purine auxotroph [reviewed in Pfefferkorn 1988]. *T. gondii* has an absolute requirement to salvage either adenosine, inosine, hypoxanthine or adenine from the host cell [Krug et al. 1989], although adenosine is the most likely substrate. Purine nucleosides and purine bases do not diffuse spontaneously across lipid bilayers, are are likely to be transported by specific transporters in the parasite plasma membrane. Transport of nucleosides across the PVM is also necessary. Although the presence of a pore within the PVM (see above) may obviate the requirement for specific purine transporters within the PVM, this hypothesis remains to be proven.

a)   Nucleoside Transport in Extracellular Tachyzoites

In work being done collaboratively with Dr Robert Handschumacher in the Department of Pharmacology at Yale University, experiments have focused initially on nucleoside transport in extracellular tachyzoites [Schwab, Handschumacher and Joiner, in prep.]. Measurement of true adenosine transport rates were initially confounded by the active intracellular phosphorylation of adenosine to nucleotide by the active parasite adenosine kinase. This problem has been circumvented, using high extracellular adenosine concentrations and an adenosine kinase deficient mutant, kindly provided by Dr Elmer Pfefferkorn. The presence of a high capacity ($Km > 400\mu M$), non-concentrative transporter has been demonstrated, with specificity for adenosine, inosine and hypoxanthine, but not other nucleosides or nucleobases.

The presence of a putative pore within the PVM of sufficient diameter to allow host cell ATP and nucleosides to readily enter the parasitophorous vacuole space suggests that selected purine salvage enzymes may be localized in the parasitophorous vacuole space. The nucleoside triphosphate hydrolase secreted from the parasite [Asai and O'Sullivan 1983; Johnson et al. 1989] should accumulate in the PV space, and under reducing conditions [Asai and Kim 1987], metabolize ATP to ADP and AMP. Further nucleoside salvage would then depend upon a secreted or membrane bound 5' nucleotidase to convert AMP to adenosine. This area is currently under investigation in our laboratory and others.

b)   Inhibition of Nucleoside Transport

Non-concentrative adenosine or inosine transport over 300 seconds in extracellular tachyzoites is completely blocked by dipyridamole ($IC_{50} = 0.8\mu M$), a non-competitive inhibitor of nucleoside transport, but blocked only 15-20% by the competitive active site inosine analogue, nitrobenzylthioinosine. This inhibition profile is distinctly different from the profile in mammalian cells [reviewed in Plagemann, et al. 1988], suggesting that specific inhibition of the parasite transport processes may be feasible.

Antibiotic uptake

Antimicrobial agents effective against *T. gondii* must enter infected cells, cross the PVM, enter the intracellular parasite and achieve sufficient concentrations at the target site to mediate antimicrobial activity. Although partial analaysis of these parameters has been completed for inhibitors of *T. gondii* folate synthesis [Allegra et al. 1987], no analogous experiments are reported with other classes of agents.

The lincosamide clindamycin, and the newer macrolides, azithromycin and clarithromycin, are bacterial protein synthesis inhibitors which are being evaluated for use as alternative therapies for *T. gondii* in patients with AIDS who fail to respond or develop adverse reactions to conventional therapy with pyrimethamine and sulfadiazine [reviewed in Remington and McLeod 1992; Dannemann 1992; Araugo, this volume; Chang, this volume]. The mechanism of action of the agents for *T. gondii* is not known. Furthermore, the activity of these agents for *T. gondii in vitro* is variable, and cannot be used to predict *in vivo* efficacy in animals or humans or to prospectively modify existing compounds based on structure-activity relationships [Chamberland et al. 1991; Harris et al. 1988; Chang and Pechere 1988]. We have undertaken experiments to study the subcellular distribution of these antibiotics within vacuoles in infected cells as part of a larger group effort [laboratories of B. Luft, D. Roos, and K. Joiner] to systematically define the mechanisms of action of the agents for *T. gondii*. The ultimate goal is the rational design of more effective agents for the treatment of *T. gondii* infections, based in part on the cell biologic aspects of intracellular *T. gondii* infection.

a) Macrolide Uptake in Infected Cells, Vacuoles and Parasites
Macrolide uptake into *T. gondii*-infected cells is rapid and concentrative, with ratios of intracellular/extracellular (I/E) drug exceeding 40:1 for azithromycin after 60 minutes at 37°C [Schwab, Cao, Beckers, Slowik and Joiner, in preparation]. Nonetheless, subcellular fractionation experiments separating parasitophorous vacuoles from cell cytosol and other cell organelles demonstrate that over 96% of intracellular azithromycin accumulates within cellular lysosomes as a consequence of protonation of the drug, which is a weak base. In contrast, less than 4% of the drug accumulates within the non-acidified parasitophorous vacuole. Of the small percentage of azithromycin which accumulates within the parasite intracellularly, the majority [>90%] is concentrated within acidifed organelles of the parasite. Hence, less than 1% of the total intracellular drug in heavily infected CHO cells localizes within the parasite cytosol or is available to bind to cytoplasmic ribosomes of the tachyzoite.

b)   Macrolides and Lincosamides: Mechanism of Action for *T. gondii*

Protein synthesis in *T. gondii* has an inhibition profile which is eukaryotic in nature [Schwab, Cao, Beckers, Slowik and Joiner, in preparation].   This suggests, in conjunction with the above results, that the mechanism of action of lincosamides and macrolides for *T. gondii* is not generalized inhibition of parasite protein synthesis.   Recent experiments from the laboratory of Dr Elmer   Pfefferkorn   (personal   communication)   suggest   indirectly   that mitochondrial ribosomes may be the target for clindamycin activity.   This is an area which is under investigation in several laboratories, including our own.

References

Allegra, C.J., Kovacs, J.A., Drake, J.C, Swan, J.C., Chabner, B.A. and Masur, H. [1987]. Potent *in vitro* and *in vivo* antitoxoplasma activity of the lipid-soluble antifolate trimetrexate. J. Clin. Invest. 79: 478-482.

Achbarou, A., Mercereau-Puijalon, O., Sadak, A., Fortier, B., Leriche, J.A., Camus, D. and Dubremetz, J.F. [1991].   Differential targeting of dense granule proteins in the parasitophorous vacuole of *Toxoplasma gondii*. Parasitology. 103: 321-329.

Asai, T. and Kim, T. [1987].   Possible regulation mechanism of potent nucleoside triphosphate hydrolase in *Toxoplasma gondii*.   Zentralbl Bakteriol Mikrobiol Hyg A. 264: 464-467.

Asai, T. and O'Sullivan, W.J. [1983].   A potent nucleoside triphosphate hydrolase from the parasitic protozoan *Toxoplasma gondii*.   J. Biol. Chem. 258: 6816-6822.

Cesbron-Delauw, M.F., Guy, B. Torpier, G., Pierce, R.J., Lenzen, G., Cesbron, J.Y., Charif, H., Lepage, P., Darcy, F., Lecocq, J.P. and Capron, A. [1989].   Molecular characterization of a 23-kilodalton major antigen secreted by *Toxoplasma gondii*.   Proc. Natl. Acad. Sci. 86: 7537-7541.

Chamberland, S., Kirst, H.A. and Current, W.L. [1991]. Comparative activity of macrolides against *Toxoplasma gondii* demonstrating utility of an *in vitro* microassay. Antimicrob. Agents Chemo. 35: 903-909.

Chang, H.R. and Pechere, J.C.F. [1988].   *In vitro* effects of four macrolides (roxithromycin, spiramycin, azithromycin [CP-62-993] and A-56268) on *Toxoplasma gondii*. Antimicrob. Agents Chemo. 32: 524-529.

Charif, H., Darcy, F., Torpier, G., Cesbron-Delauw, M.F. and Capron, A. [1990]. "Characterization and localization of antigens secreted from tachyzoites. Exp. Parasit. 71: 114-124.

Danneman, B. [1992]. Treatment of toxoplasmic encephalitis in patients with AIDS: A randomized trial comparing pyrimethamine plus clindamycin to pyrimethamine plus sulfadiazine. Ann. Int. Med. 116: 33-43.

Furtado, G.C., Slowik, M., Kleinman, H.K. and Joiner, K.A. [1992c]. Laminin enhances binding of *Toxoplasma gondii* tachyzoites to J774 murine macrophage cells. Infect. Immun. 60: 2337-2342.

Furtado, G.C., Collins, F.L., Cao, J. and Joiner, K.A., [1992a]. Laminin on tachyzoites of *Toxoplasma gondii* mediates parasite binding to the $\beta 1$ integrin receptor $\alpha 6 \beta 1$ on human foreskin fibroblasts and Chinese hamster ovary cells. Submitted:

Furtado, G.C., Fuhrman, S.A., Dubremetz, J.F. and Joiner, K.A. [1992b]. Detergent insolube surface proteins on *Toxoplasma gondii* mediate cell attachment and include host-derived laminin and 32/67 laminin binding protein. Submitted:

Harris, C., Salgo, M.P. Tanowitz, H.B., and Wittner, M. [1988] *In vitro* assessment of antimicrobial agents against *Toxoplasma gondii*. J. Infect. Dis. 157: 14-22.

Johnson, A.M., Illana, S., McDonald, P.J., and Asai, T. [1989]. Cloning expression and nucleotide sequence of the gene fragment encoding an antigenic portion of the nucleoside triphosphate hydrolase of *Toxoplasma gondii*. Gene. 85: 215-220.

Joiner, K.A., Fuhrman, S.A., Mietinnen, H., Kasper, L.H., and Mellman, I. [1990]. *Toxoplasma gondii*: Fusion competence of parasitophorous vacuoles in Fc receptor transfected fibroblasts. Science. 249: 641-646.

Jones, T.C. and Hirsch, J.G. [1972]. The interaction between *Toxoplasma gondii* and mammalian cells. II. The absence of lysosomal fusion with phagocytic vacuoles containing living parasites. J. Exp. Med. 136: 1173.

Krug, E.C., Marr, J.J. and Berens, R.L. [1989]. Purine metabolism in *Toxoplasma gondii*. J. Biol. Chem. 264: 10601-10607.

Leriche, M.A. and Dubremetz, J.F. [1991]. Characterization of the protein contents of rhoptries and dense granules of *Toxoplasma gondii* tachyzoites by subcellular fractionation and monoclonal antibodies. Mol. Biochem. Parasit. 45: 249-260.

Pfefferkorn, E.R. [1988]. *Toxoplasma gondii* viewed from a virological perspective. The Biology of Parasitism., New York, Alan R. Liss.

Plagemann, P.G.W., Wohlhueter, R.M. and Woffendin, C. [1988]. Nucleoside and nucleobase transport in animal cells. Biochim. Biophys. Acta. 947: 405-443.

Porchet-Hennere, E. and Torpier, G. [1983]. Relations entre *Toxoplasma* et sa cellule-hote. Protistologica. 3: 357.

Remington, J.S. and McLeod, R. [1992]. Toxoplasmosis. Infectious Diseases. Philadelphia, W.B. Saunders.

Sibley, D.L. and Krahenbuhl, J.L. [1988]. Modification of host cell phagosomes by *Toxoplasma gondii* involves redistribution of surface proteins and secretion of a 32kDa protein. Eur. J. Cell Biol. 47: 81-87.

Sibley, L.D., Krahenbuhl, J.L., Adams, G.M.W. and Weidner, E. [1986]. *Toxoplasma* modifies macrophage phagosomes by secretion of a vesicular network rich in surface proteins. J. Cell Biol. 103: 867-874.

Sibley, L.D., Weidner, E. and Krahenbuhl, J.L. [1985]. Phagosome acidification blocked by intracellular *Toxoplasma gondii*. Nature. 315: 1985.

Werk, R. [1985]. How does *Toxoplasma gondii* enter host cells? Rev. Infect. Dis. 7: 449-457.

TOXOPLASMA GONDII MOTILITY AND INVASION

J. D. Schwartzman*
Department of Pathology
University of Virginia Health Sciences Center
Charlottesville, VA 22908

Host cell penetration by *Toxoplasma gondii*, as observed *in vitro* by light microscopy of cultured cell monolayers, is a rapid process quite distinct from phagocytosis. Active parasite processes including gliding motility, shape changes mediated by the parasite cytoskeleton, the formation of a moving junction with the host plasma membrane, the secretion of factors from parasite organelles, and the formation of a specialized intracellular vacuole (in which the parasite resides and that does not fuse with host lysosomes) are all important to successful host cell penetration and intracellular survival. Parasite motility is a primary effector of invasion, since *T. gondii* immobilized by various means does not get inside most host cells. The process of attachement and penetration seems to feature considerable redundancy, which allows *T. gondii* to invade and parasitize a wide variety of hosts.

Morphology of Invasion

The basic behaviour of *T. gondii* in its interaction with cells in culture has been observed by light microscopy [Bogatchev, et al. 1980; Bommer, et al. 1969; Doran 1973; Hirai, et al. 1966]. Saltatory gliding motility of tachyzoites over a solid substrate is followed by rapid penetration in cultured cells of almost any type. The movement of the parasite is in a forward clockwise "corkscrew" fashion without obvious deformation of the parasite body, although torsion of the parasite external membrane has been noted by scanning electronmicroscopy [Aikawa, et al. 1977; Chiappino, et al. 1984]. Anterior-posterior flexing of non-gliding parasites and forward protrusion of the anterior tip of the organism can also be seen.

---

* Present address: Department of Pathology, Dartmouth-Hitchcock Medical Center, Lebanon, New Hampshire 03756 USA

NATO ASI Series, Vol. H 78
Toxoplasmosis
Edited by Judith E. Smith
© Springer-Verlag Berlin Heidelberg 1993

Although motility is a key part of the process of active penetration in *Toxoplasma* the mechanism has never been explained. Evidence for the central role of parasite motility in host cell penetration is provided by the observation that parasites transiently immobilized by low temperature, change of pH, change of extracellular ion milieu, or by reversible inhibitors of cytoskeletal function such as cytochalasins, are unable to enter host cells, but regain their ability to invade when the inhibiting factor is removed [Doran 1973; Endo and Yagita 1990; Russell and Sinden 1981; Schwartzman and Pfefferkorn 1983]. Parasite metabolic energy [Werk and Bommer 1980] and also perhaps host metabolic energy [Kimata and Tanabe 1982; Kimata, et al. 1987] is required for host cell invasion.

Gliding movement similar to that of *T. gondii* is seen in bacteria, fungi, algae and other protozoa, but it is not well understood in any system [Bloodgood 1989]. The transport of particles attached to the surface of algal flagellae along tracks defined by submembranous microtubules [Bloodgood 1977; Bloodgood 1981] presents one promising model of gliding locomotion; another that has been suggested is the capping of ligands such as antibody molecules on cell surfaces. Free-living gregarine sporozoans are the organisms most closely related to *Toxoplasma* in which locomotion has been studied [King 1981; King 1988]. Like *Toxoplasma*, the gregarines only move when the organism is in contact with a substratum. In this system inhibitors of actin/myosin and calmodulin block motility [King and Lee 1982].

The question of what component *Toxoplasma* interacts with as it glides across a cell surface or solid substrate, or as it invades a host cell is unclear. It has been suggested that laminin may have an important role in this regard [Furtado, et al. 1992; Joiner, et al. 1989] but other molecules may also function in this role. The role of *Toxoplasma* surface antigens or secreted factors in this process needs to be defined. *Plasmodium* and *Eimeria* sporozoites appear to leave trails of circumsporozoite protein on solid substrates over which they have moved [Entzeroth, et al. 1989; Stewart and Vandenberg 1988], which could be related to their mode of locomotion, and raises the question of whether *Toxoplasma gondii* surface antigens could play a similar role. A protein has recently been described in malaria that may have a role in forming the moving junction seen in the invasion of the merozoite into the erythrocyte [Klotz, et al. 1989]. No such molecule has been defined in *Toxoplasma*.

Possible motors

Toxoplasma and *Eimeria* are made immotile by low concentrations of Cytochalasin D [King 1988; Ryning and Remington 1978; Schwartzman and Pfefferkorn 1983], an agent that interferes with actin polymerization and interrupts microfilament based motility in a number of eukaryotic systems [Goddette and Frieden 1986]. This is not direct proof that actin/myosin interactions are responsible for *T. gondii* motility because cytochalasins have been shown to have other actions including interference with glucose transport. The effect of cytochalasin at concentrations at which its predominant effect is on actin [Ohmori, et al. 1992], combined with the evidence that most whole cell locomotion in eukaryotes is powered by actin/myosin [Small 1989], favours myosin as the motor powering *T. gondii* gliding.

Actin/myosin has been implicated in the mechanism of motility of gregarine sporozoans. Actin is localized at the internal cytomembranes and in the cortical ectoplasm of gregarines [Baines and King 1989b]. By western immunoblot using anti-actin antibody, both the expected 43 kDa protein and a higher molecular weight species were detected in gregarines and in *Eimeria* [Baines and King 1989a; Baines and King 1989b]. We have studied the distribution and organization of myosin and tubulin in *T. gondii* by immunofluorescence microscopy utilizing antibodies specific for cytoskeletal proteins of heterologous organisms [Schwartzman, et al. 1985; Schwartzman and Pfefferkorn 1983]. Myosin appears to be concentrated at the anterior pole of *T. gondii*. Actin appeared uniformly distributed in our studies (unpublished results) either in the cytoplasm or perhaps associated with membranes, but not organized into filaments. Endo has reported that actin is localized to the anterior of *T. gondii* [Endo, et al. 1988; Yasuda, et al. 1988], and Taylor et al. [1990] have found an antigen in many sporozoans which has an anterior distribution, and which they suspect may be actin. Two actin genes of malaria have recently been cloned and sequenced, and it is of interest that one of the two genes displays the most divergent sequence of any actin gene so far studied [Wesseling, et al. 1988a; Wesseling, et al. 1988b]. No myosin genes have been cloned from parasitic protozoa, but both classical (myosin II) and small (myosin I) myosins have been described in *Acanthamoeba* and *Dictyostelium* [Korn and Hammer 1988]. Some myosin I isoforms have been found to be membrane associated, and may be implicated in whole cell locomotion [Fukui, et al. 1989; Miyata, et al. 1989].

There are multiple myosin-like motors that interact with actin to power numerous intracellular tasks [Spudich 1989]. *Toxoplasma* would be expected to have both myosin types. Myosin is, in general, less conserved in total amino acid sequence than other cytosketletal proteins, but contains strongly conserved regions, especially in the globular head, associated with the ATP and actin binding sites [Korn, et al. 1988; Titus, et al. 1989]. The tail regions of myosins are much more diverse, correlating with specialization of intracellular function [Korn and Hammer 1988].

Tubulin-based motility may be important in some phase of *T. gondii* invasion. The distribution of tubulin in *T. gondii* corresponds to the described subpellicular microtubules, and the conoid [Schwartzman, et al. 1985]. Tubulin has been cloned from *T. gondii*, and is 80-90% identical in amino acid sequence in both alpha and beta subunits compared to tubulin from diverse taxa [Nagel and Boothroyd 1988].

Mechanism of Gliding

Understanding the mechanism of gliding locomotion in *T. gondii* is complicated by the unusual arrangement of membranes of *T. gondii* zoites. An apparently ordinary plasma membrane surrounds the organism. Two additional unit membranes have been noted internal to the plasma membrane, which have been shown in *Eimeria* and *Sarcocystis* [Porchet-Hennere 1975] to be arranged as side-by-side envelopes appearing like "pavement blocks", with cross sections showing two unit membranes closely opposed. Freeze facture micrographs [Schwartzman and Saffer 1992] demonstrate similar patches of inner membrane complex in *T. gondii*. The somewhat irregular "blocks" are not continuous over the surface of the tachyzoite: the inner membrane complex is absent at the poles of the organism. Beneath the inner membrane complex are the cytoplasm and 22 pairs of longitudinal microtubules [Nichols and Chiappino 1987]. If the outer membrane must be coupled to a surface in order to transduce force, and if the motor is located in the cytoplasm, the inner membrane complex is interposed. Transmembrane glycoproteins have been shown to couple microtubule-associated motors to external ligands in *Chlamydomonas* flagella [Bloodgood and Salomonsky 1989]. The multiple membrane layers of sporozoans would appear to complicate such a scheme of parasite motility. The simplest model would place the motor proteins beneath the outer membrane of the parasite. Transmembrane proteins would be required to couple the motor to the substrate, but no transmembrane protein of *T. gondii* has yet been described, the major surface proteins are all thought to be glycolipid anchored [Nagel and Boothroyd 1989; Tomavo, et al. 1989].

Control of Motility

The initiation of *T. gondii* motility has been reported to be stimulated by changes in the internal pH and K+ concentration, as studied by the use of the fluorescent weak base 9-amino acridine [Endo, et al. 1987]. Acidification of the external medium can induce motility in extracellular parasites. Manipulation of the extracellular pH and ionic milieu can temporarily immobilize extracellular *Toxoplasma* [Endo and Yagita 1990]. The calcium ionophore A23187 induces motility in intracellular *T. gondii* [Endo, et al. 1982]. The calmodulin inhibitor trifluoperizine inhibits gliding motility in gregarine sporozoans [King and Lee 1982], but does not affect motility of *T. gondii* (Schwartzman, unpublished results). The interaction of ions in the initiation of motility of *Toxoplasma* remains to be elucidated.

Strategies for the Study of Motility and Invasiveness

Understanding the mechanism of *Toxoplasma gondii* motility in relation to host cell invasion may allow the design of strategies to interrupt both acute toxoplasmosis and the reactivation of latent toxoplasmosis. Useful steps toward this goal include characterization of *T. gondii* myosin, a candidate for the primary motor protein powering gliding motility. Extraction and biochemical study of the native protein is limited by the difficulty of obtaining sufficient organisms, and by contamination with host cell protein. It should be possible to study the parasite protein by cloning and sequencing the *T. gondii* myosin gene(s) for comparison of primary sequence with functional domains of known myosin genes. Expression of the parasite myosin gene would allow analysis of the biochemical and functional properties of the molecule. It will also be useful to produce specific antibodies for morphological and immunochemical studies of myosin distribution, stage specific expression and function.

A complementary approach to the study of motility and invasiveness is selection of mutant strains of *T. gondii* for the study of motility and cytosketletal function in host cell invasion. Selection of mutant strains resistant to pharmacological agents affecting assembly or function of cytoskeletal proteins, or of mutant strains with conditional alterations of motility or invasiveness will allow analysis of the phenotype and virulence of the mutant parasites and correlation of the mutations with genotype. An understanding of the interactions of the parasite cytoskeleton which result in gliding motility will provide a novel target for the interruption of *Toxoplasma* pathogenesis.

References

Aikawa M, Komata Y, Asai T, Midorikawa, O (1977) Transmission and scanning electron microscopy of host cell entry by *Toxoplasma gondii*. Am. J. Pathol. 87: 285-296.

Baines I, King, C A (1989a) Demonstration of actin in sporozoites of the protozoon *Eimeria*. Cell Biol. Internat. Rep. 13: 639-641.

Baines I, King, C A (1989b) Demonstration of actin in the protozoon *Gregarina*. Cell Biol. Internat. Rep. 13: 679-686.

Bloodgood, R A (1977) Motility occurring in association with the surface of the *Chlamydomonas* flagellum. J. Cell Biol. 75: 983-989.

Bloodgood, R A (1981) Flagellum as a model system for studying dynamic cell-surface events. Cold Spring Harbor Symp. Quant. Biol. 46: 683-693.

Bloodgood, R A (1989) Gliding motility: can regulated protein movements in the plasma membrane drive whole cell locomotion? Cell Motil. Cytoskel. 14: 340-344.

Bloodgood, R A, Salomonsky, N L (1989) Use of a novel *Chlamydomonas* mutant to demonstrate that flagellar glycoprotein movements are necessary for the expression of gliding motility. Cell Motil. Cytoskel. 13: 1-8.

Bogatchev, Y V, Khavkin, T N, Shustrov, A K, Freidlin, I S (1980) Motion picture study of the response of cultured peritoneal macrophages to the invasion of endozoits of *Toxoplasma gondii*, RH strain. Acta Microbiol. Acad. Sci. Hung. 27: 1-8.

Bommer W, Heunert, H H, Milthaler, B (1969) Cinematographic studies on the movement of *Toxoplasma gondii*. Z. Tropenmed. Parasitol. 20: 450-8.

Chiappino M L, Nichols B A, O'Connor G R (1984) Scanning electron microscopy of *Toxoplasma gondii*: parasite torsion and host-cell responses during invasion. J. Protozool. 31: 288-92.

Doran D J, (1973) Cultivation of Coccidia in avian embryos and cell culture. In The Coccidia: *Eimeria, Isopora, Toxoplasma*, and related genera. University Park Press, Baltimore.

Endo T, Sethi K K, Piekarski, G (1982) *Toxoplasma gondii*: Calcium ionophore A23187-mediated exit of trophozoites from infected murine macrophages. Exp. Parasitol. 53: 179-188.

Endo T, Tokuda H, Yagita K, Koyama T (1987) Effects of extracellular potassium on acid release and motility initiation in *Toxoplasma gondii*. J. Protozool. 34: 291-295.

Endo T, Yagita K (1990) Effect of extracellular ions on motility and cell entry in *Toxoplasma gondii*. J. Protozool. 37: 133-138.

Endo T, Yagita K, Yasuda T, Nakamura T (1988) Detection and localization of actin in *Toxoplasma gondii*. Parasitol. Res. 75: 102-106.

Entzeroth R, Zgrzebski, G, Dubremetz J F (1989) Secretion of trails during gliding motility of *Eimeria nieschulzi* (Apicomplexa, Coccidia) sporozoites visualized by a monoclonal antibody and immuno-gold-silver enhancement. Parasitol. Res. 76: 174-5.

Fukui Y, Lynch T J, Brzeska H, Korn ED (1989) Myosin 1 is located at the leading edges of locomoting *Dictyostelium* amoebae. Nature 341: 328-331.

Furtado G C, Slowik M, Kleinman HK, Joiner K A (1992) Laminin enhances binding of *Toxoplasma gondii* tachyzoites to J774 murine macrophage cells. Infect. Immun. 60: 2337-2342.

Goddette D W, Frieden C (1986) Actin polymerization. The mechanism of action of cytochalasin D. J. Biol.Chem. 261: 15974-15980.

Hirai K, Hirato K, Yanagwa R (1966) A cinematographic study of the penetration of cultured cells by *Toxoplasma gondii*. Jpn. J. Vet. Res. 14: 81-90.

Joiner K A, Furtado G, Mellman I, Kleinman H, Miettinen H, Kasper L, Hall L, Fuhrman S (1989) Cell attachment and invasion by tachyzoites of *Toxoplasma gondii*. J. Cell Biochem. Suppl. 13: 64.

Kimata I, Tanabe K (1982) Invasion by *Toxoplasma gondii* of ATP-depleted and ATP-restored chick embryo erythrocytes. J. Gen. Microbiol. 128: 2499-2501.

Kimata I, Tanabe K, Izumo A, Takada S (1987) Host cell ATP level and invasion of *Toxoplasma gondii*. Trans. Royal Soc. Trop. Med. Hyg. 81: 377.

King C A (1981) Cell surface interaction of the protozoan *Gregarina* with Concanavalin A beads - implications for models of gregarine gliding. Cell Biol. Int. Rep. 5: 297.

King C A (1988) Cell motility of sporozoan protozoa. Parasitol. Today 4: 315-319.

King C A, Lee K (1982) Effect of trifluoperazine and calcium ions on gregarine gliding. Experientia. 38: 1051-1052.

Klotz F W, Hadley T J, Aikawa M, Leech J, Howard R J, Miller L H (1989) A 60-kDa *Plasmodium falciparum* protein at the moving junction formed between merozoite and erythrocyte during invasion. Mol Biochem. Parasitol. 36: 177-85.

Korn E D, Atkinson M A L, Brzeska H, Hammer J A, Jung G, Lynch T L (1988) Structure-Function Studies on *Acanthamoeba* Myosins 1A, 1B, and 11. J. Cell Biochem. 36: 37-50.

Korn E D, Hammer J A (1988) Myosins of nonmuscle cells. Annu. Rev. Biophys. Chem. 17: 23-45.

Miyata H, Bowers B, Korn E D (1989) Plasma membrane association of *Acanthamoeba* myosin 1. J. Cell Biol. 109: 1519-1528.

Nagel S D, Boothroyd J C (1988) The alpha- and beta-tubulins of *Toxoplasma gondii* are encoded by single copy genes containing multiple introns. Molec. Biochem. Parasit. 29: 261-273.

Nagel S D, Boothroyd J C (1989) The major surface antigen, P30, of *Toxoplasma gondii* is anchored by a glycolipid. J. Cell Biol. 264: 5569-5574.

Nichols B A, Chiappino M L (1987) Cytoskeleton of *Toxoplasma gondii*. J. Protozool. 34: 217-226.

Ohmori H, Toyama S, Toyama S (1992) Direct proof that the primary site of action of Cytochalasin on cell motility is actin. J. Cell Biol. 116: 933-941.

Porchet-Hennere E (1975) Quelques précisions sur l'ultrastructure de *Sarcocystis tenella*. L'endozoite (aprés coloration negative) J. Protozool. 22: 214-220.

Russell D G, Sinden R E (1981) The role of the cytoskeleton in the motility of Coccidian sporozoites. J. Cell Sci. 50: 345-359.

Ryning F W, Remington J S (1978) Effect of cytochalasin D on *Toxoplasma gondii* cell entry. Infect. Immun. 20: 739-743.

Schwartzman J D, Krug E C, Payne M R Binder L I (1985) Detection of the microtubule cytoskeleton of the Coccidian *Toxoplasma gondii* and the hemoflagellate *Leishmania donovani* by monoclonal antibodies specific for beta-tubulin. J. Protozool. 32: 747-749.

Schwartzman J D, Pfefferkorn E R (1983) Immunofluorescent localization of myosin at the anterior pole of the Coccidian, *Toxoplasma gondii*. J. Protozool. 30: 657-661.

Schwartzman J D, Saffer L D (1992) How *Toxoplasma gondii* gets in and out of cells. Subcellular Biochemistry: 18. In Intracellular Parasites Avila and Haris (eds) Plenum Publishing Corporation, New York.

Small J V (1989) Microfilament-based motility in non-mucle cells. Curr. Opin. Cell Biol. 1: 75-79.

Spudich J A (1989) In pursuit of myosin function. Cell Regulation 1: 1-11.

Stewart M J, Vandenberg J P (1988) Malaria sporozoites leave behind trails of circumsporozite protein during gliding motility. J. Protozool. 35: 389-393.

Taylor D W, Evans CB, Aley S B, Barta J R, Danforth H D (1990) Identification of an apically-located antigen that is conserved in sporozoan parasites. J. Protozool. 37: 540-545.

Titus M A, Warrick H A, Spudich J A (1989) Multiple actin-based motor genes in *Dictyostelium*. Cell Regulation 1: 55-63.

Tomavo S, Schwarz R T, Dubremetz J F (1989) Evidence for glycosyl-phosphatidylinositol anchoring of *Toxoplasma gondii* major surface antigens. Mol. Cell Bio. 9: 4576-80.

Werk R, Bommer W (1980) *Toxoplasma gondii*: Membrane properties of active energy-dependent invasion of host cells. Tropenmed. Parasitol. 31: 417-420.

Wesseling J G, de Ree J M, Ponnudurai T, Smits M A, Schoenmakers J G G (1988a) Nucleotide Sequence and deduced amino acid sequence of a *Plasmodium falciparum* actin gene. Molec. Biochem. Parasitol. 27: 313-320.

Wesseling J G, Smits M A, Schoenmakers J G G (1988b) Extremely diverged actin proteins in *Plasmodium falciparum*. Molec. Biochem. Parasitol. 30: 143-154.

Yasuda T, Yagita K, Nakamura T, Endo T (1988) Immunocytochemical localization of actin in *Toxoplasma gondii*. Parasitol. Res. 75: 107-113.

TOXOPLASMA GONDII: PATTERNS OF BRADYZOITE-TACHYZOITE INTERCONVERSION IN VITRO

Martine Soete,, Bernard Fortier, Daniel Camus and Jean Francois Dubremetz
INSERM Unite 42
369 rue Jules Guesde
59 650 Villeneuve d'Ascq

The development of *Toxoplasma gondii* in the intermediate host is believed to be a balance between the parasite and the immune system of the host which leads to either of the two possible developmental stages that are tachyzoites or bradyzoites. Alteration of the balance leads to interconversion between these stages [Frenkel et al, 1975]. The relations between the immune response and the mechanism(s) of interconversion are unknown. Since analyzing these phenomena in the host is complex, we have started investigating this phenomenon *in vitro*. We have confirmed the previous description by others of strains producing both stages *in vitro* in the absence of any immunological effector [Hoff et al, 1977; Darde et al, 1989]. This system will be used to characterize the essential requirements for differentiation toward either of the two stages. The strategy developed towards this goal is as follows: first to obtain stages specific probes; second to follow spontaneous differentiation *in vitro*, and third to find ways of manipulating differentiation in order to define the mechanisms involved. The first two steps will be described in this report.

Stage specific probes and structures

Recent studies have shown that mixed populations of organisms expressing tachyzoite or bradyzoite specific molecules, or both, occur simultaneously *in vitro*. The references we used for defining specificity are tachyzoites grown in the peritoneal cavity of mice and bradyzoites obtained from cysts grown in mice brain.

Stage specific probes: Tachyzoite specific monoclonal antibodies (MAbs) were obtained several years ago [Handman et al, 1980], although their lack of reactivity with bradyzoites was only clearly established recently. These are anti P30 and anti P22 (SAG 1; SAG 2). They recognize surface proteins, GPI anchored in the tachyzoite membrane. Other surface molecules such as P43 (SAG 3) or P23 (SAG 4) are common to tachyzoites and bradyzoites.

NATO ASI Series, Vol. H 78
Toxoplasmosis
Edited by Judith E. Smith
© Springer-Verlag Berlin Heidelberg 1993

Bradyzoite specific Mabs have been developed more recently [Omata et al, 1989; Tomavo et al, 1991]. The target molecules are not fully characterized yet, due to the difficulty in obtaining enough material for study. Apart from the 20 kDa described as internal [Omata et al, 1989], the four others (BAG1 or Pb21, BAG2 or Pb36, BAG3 or Pb34 and BAG4 or Pb18) have been localized in the pellicle, three of them being accessible either to antibodies or to trypsin cleavage, or both, and likely to be surface located [Tomavo et al, 1991]. The way they are anchored in the membrane remains to be investigated. All the probes specific for organelles (rhoptries, micronemes, dense granules) that we have tested so far were common to both stages and therefore cannot be used for studying differentiation. They may have some interest however, since variation in the abundance of organelles (such as micronemes) or in targetting of the contents (for dense granules, see below) may occur with developmental stage.

Stage specific structure : Tachyzoites are typically found in vacuoles, bradyzoites are found in cysts: these are two ways for the parasite to create a new compartment in the host cell. The parasitophorous vacuole containing tachyzoites has a single membrane connected with a well developed intravacuolar tubular network. Both the vacuole membrane and the network are associated with proteins exocytosed from the dense granules of the tachyzoites [Achbarou et al, 1991]. Bradyzoites are typically found in a cyst which is originally found with a cell, even though this association has sometimes been questioned in later stages. The cyst wall is more complex but is also bound by a single membrane with irregular invaginations and an underlying layer of homogenous osmiophilic material [Ferguson et al, 1987a]. When compared to the parasitophorous vacuole, cyst formation can be considered as the development of a new compartment having a different system of exchange with the host cell: the cyst cannot be a closed system but is probably less active metabolically since cysts grow in size and bradyzoites multiply inside.

Therefore, the switch between stages should trigger both the synthesis of new molecules on zoites and a different pattern of interaction with the host cell; building a different compartment may involve a different pattern of exocytosis, or a different content of dense granules, as those identified so far are the major contributors to the development of the parasitophorous vacuole in the tachyzoite stage.

Differentiation *in vitro*

We have followed the spontaneous switches that occur when inoculating cell cultures with parasites obtained from mice. We used the following strains: Strain BQNC2 was recently isolated from a human infection, used to infect mouse, multiplied *in vitro* and cloned by limited dilution (B. Fortier; unpublished); Strain 76K has been isolated from a guinea pig [Laugier and Quilici, 1970] and is routinely used as chronic strain in the laboratory; Strain Prugniaud was isolated from a case of human lethal congenital toxoplasmosis [Martrou et al, 1965]. We used four MAb specific for bradyzoite proteins: Pb36 (T8 4A12), Pb34 (T8 2C2), Pb21 (T8 4G10) and Pb18 (T8 3B1) [Tomavo et al, 1991] and one MAb specific for a tachyzoite surface protein: SAG1 (P30: T4 1E5) [Couvreur et al, 1988].

Differentiation of bradyzoite into tachyzoite : When bradyzoites obtained from brain cysts (strain 76K or BQNC2) invade a cell monolayer (Vero cells), one finds no antigenic changes for about 15 h after invasion, i.e. all four bradyzoite specific molecules are found, but no SAG1. At 15 hours post infection (p.i.), we observed intermediate stages which were doubly labelled and expressed SAG1 in addition to bradyzoite specific molecules. At about 24 hours p.i. the division of parasites began; we could observe the multiplication of the intermediate stages. At 48 hours p.i., we observed more multiplication of doubly labelled parasites and also organisms which had completely lost bradyzoite specific determinants and which we therefore considered to be tachyzoites. The relative number of doubly labelled parasites decreased during the course of the experiment, due to disapearance of bradyzoite specific protein expression and to the multiplication of tachyzoites which diluted the other stages. Multiplication of bradyzoites started at around 48 hours p.i. for BQNC2 strain and at around 72 hours p.i. for 76K strain: small vacuoles containing several organisms which did not react with anti-SAG1 were found at these respective times in both strains.

Infection of cells with bradyzoites (strain BQNC2) resulted in the generation of heterogenous parasitophorous vacuoles at 72 hours p.i. Indeed, within a single parsitophorous vacuole, we found parasites expressing different levels of bradyzoite or tachyzoite molecules. These vacuoles usually contained intermediate organisms mixed together with P30 negative or positive parasites.

Differentiation of tachyzoite into bradyzoite : Tachyzoites of the Prugniaud strain harvested from the peritoneal cavity of mice did not react with bradyzoite specific MAb, but expressed SAG1. At 24 hours p.i., we observed essentially tachyzoites which were dividing and a low percentage of parasites reacting faintly with three of the four bradyzoite specific MAbs (anti P36, P34 and P18), At 48 hours p.i., we observed typical doubly labelled parasites which were dividing, although the tachyzoites were still a large majority, however no parasites reacted with the anti P21 antibody. At 72 hours p.i., organisms which had completely lost the tachyzoite specific determinant began to appear. Heterogenous vacuoles similar to those observed during BQNC2 transformation were also found, but there was still no reactivity with P21.

Stage specific molecules expressed during permanent culture in vitro : When chronic strains such as BQNC" or 76K or Prugniaud are maintained in cell monolayers, all stages are permanently found simultaneously in the culture, but what changes is the relative number of parasites which express either only tachyzoites or bradyzoite specific molecules or both. P21 is always found less frequently than the other bradyzoite specific proteins. Variations in the relative abundance of stages found in a culture could not be clearly related to any chamical or physical parameter. Episodes of slow multiplication in which most of the zoites would develop slowly and express bradyzoite specific proteins alternate with outgrowth of tachyzoites that could eventually destroy the monolayer but could also return to slow multiplication upon transfer to another flask of cells. Vacuoles containing different stages could be found in a single cell, which suggests that stage specific expression is not permanently controlled by the host cell condition.
Preliminary data suggest that the metabolic condition of the host cell is a key factor in differentiation : tachyzoites would develop when cells are in optimal growth conditions whereas bradyzoite formation would occur when cells are faced with deleterious conditions. One major question remains as to whether differentiation is triggered upon invasion or later. Indeed, one can wonder

whether invasion always leads to a typical vacuole first, followed by later adaptation depending on what type of differentiation is switched intracellulary, or whether bradyzoites could make a different type of compartment upon invasion, which would immediately behave as a cyst. All existing data on *in vivo* cyst formation [Ferguson et al, 1987b] as well as our results *in vivo* suggest that a tachyzoite vacuole occurs first and can then transform into a cyst. Such a transformation is likely to be irreversible, and a cyst would not return to a vacuole. As suggested above, this implies that the intracellular environment would be responsible for driving the development of the parasite towards the bradyzoite or tachyzoite development. It also means that even though this environment could change, commitment to bradyzoite cannot be reversed. This would explain why we could find both stages within the same cell, since a cell containing a developing cyst could still be invaded and support tachyzoite growth. It does not explain why we observe mixed vacuoles, which remains a puzzling issue.

Conclusion

Stage specific probes allow a detailed analysis at the molecular level of bradyzoite-tachyzoite interconversion *in vitro*. This study opens up the experimental manipulation of this interconversion by modifying culture parameters. Whether the conditions that drive interconversion *in vitro* mimic events occuring under immune pressure *in vivo* will then need to be evaluated. These investigations will eventually lead to a better control of toxoplasmic reactivation, which is one of the major causes of central nervous system infection in AIDS patients.

Acknowledgments:

This work was funded by INSERM and CNRS and Agence Nationale de Recherche sur le SIDA (ANRS).

References

Achbarou, A., Mercereau-Puijalon, O., Sadak, A., Fortier, B., Leriche, M.A., Camus, D., Dubremetz, J.F., [1991] Differential targeting of dense granule proteins in the parasitophorous vacuole of *Toxoplasma gondii*. Parasitol. 103: 321-329.

Couvreur, G., Sadak, A., Fortier, B., Dubremetz, J.F. [1988] Surface antigens of *Toxoplasma gondii*. Parasitol. 97: 1-10.

Darde, M.L., Bouteille, B., Leboutet, M.J., Loubet. A., Pestre-Alexandre, M. [1989] *Toxoplasma gondii*: étude ultrastructurale des formations kystiques observées en culture de fibroblastes humans. Ann Parasitol. Hum. Comp. 64: 403-411.

Ferguson, D.J.P., Hutchison, W.M. [1987a] The hose parasite relationship of *Toxoplasma gondii* in the brain of chronically infected mice. Virchows. Arch. 411: 39-43.

Ferguson, D.J.P., Hutchison, W.M. [1987b] An ultrstructural study of the early development and tissue cyst formation of *Toxoplasma gondii* in the brains of mice. Parasitol. Res. 73: 483-491.

Frenkel, J.K., Nelson, B.M., Arias-Stella, J. [1975] Immunosuppression and toxoplasmic encephalitis. Hum. Pathol. 6: 97-111.

Handman, E., Goding, J.W., Remington. J.S. [1980] Detection and characterization of membrane antigens of *Toxoplasma gondii*. J. Immunol. 124: 2578-2583.

Hoff, R.L., Dubey, J.P., Frenkel, J.K. [1977] *Toxoplasma gondii* cysts in cell culture: new biologic evidence. J. Parasitol. 63: 1121-1124.

Laugier, M.N., Uilici, M. [1970] Interêt experimental d'une souche de toxoplasme peu pathogène pour la souris. Ann. Parasitol. Hum. Comp. 45: 389-403.

Martrou, P., Pestre-Alexandre, M., Loubet, R., Nicholas, J.A., Malinvaud, G.[1965] La toxoplasmose congénitale (note concernant un cas mortel) Limousin Medical 53: 3-7.

Omata, Y., Igarashi, M., Ramos, M.I., Nakabayashi, T. [1989] *Toxoplasma gondii*: antigenic differences between endozoites and cystozoites defined by monoclonal antibodies. Parasitol. Res. 75: 189-193.

Tomavo, S., Fortier, B., Soete, M., Ansel, C., Camus, D., Dubremetz, J.F. [1991] Characterization of bradyzoite - specific antigens of *Toxoplasma gondii*. Infect. Immun. 59: 3750-3753.

THE GROWTH AND DEVELOPMENT OF *TOXOPLASMA GONDII* TISSUE CYSTS *IN VITRO.*

Judith E. Smith & Emma K.Lewis*
Department of Pure & Applied Biology
University of Leeds
Leeds, LS29JT
UK

Like many protozoan parasites *Toxoplasma gondii* has a complex life cycle involving both sexual and asexual reproduction. In intermediate hosts the parasite exists in two distinct stages; the proliferative tachyzoite, responsible for dissemination of the parasite through host tissues during the early acute phase of infection, and the bradyzoite which forms persistent tissue cysts in brain and muscle. Conversion between these two forms appears to be reversible and is a major factor in both limiting the extent of the acute phase infection and in recrudescence of the disease, which leads to fatal toxoplasmic encephalitis in AIDS patients [Luft & Remington 1988].

Despite strong similarities in the structure of bradyzoites and tachyzoites, Western blot analysis has shown that the two stages are antigenically distinct [Kasper 1989, Woodison & Smith 1990]. Protein profiles [Zhang & Smith subm] and isoenzymes [Darde this volume] differ and molecules specific to tachyzoites [Kasper *et al* ., 1983] and to bradyzoites [Omata *et al* ., 1989, Tomavo *et al.*, 1991, Weiss *et al.*, 1992, Zhang & Smith subm] have been identified. These changes must reflect underlying differences in metabolism between the two stages.

The tachyzoite is relatively well understood both at the cellular and the molecular level. Groups of proteins on the parasite surface [Couvreur *et al* ., 1988] and in dense granules, rhoptries and micronemes have been identified [Leriche & Dubremetz 1991 Achbarou *et al* ., 1991] and several molecules have been cloned and sequenced [Burg *et al* ., 1988, Cesbron-Delauw *et al* ., 1989, Ossorio *et al.,* 1992].

In comparison much less is known about the tissue cyst. Biochemical studies rely on mature cysts harvested from experimental animals and the early growth and development of the cyst remains poorly characterized. This is largely because developing cysts are not readily accesible *in vivo* and a reliable *in ·vitro* culture system is required. Sucessful growth of tissue cysts has been reported by several authors, under widely differing conditions [Hoff *et al* ., 1977, Jones *et al* ., 1986, Lindsay *et al* .,1991] but no quantitative assessments of

---

* Now at: International Institute of Biophysics & Genetics, Via Marconi 10,
80125 Naples, Italy.

NATO ASI Series, Vol. H 78
Toxoplasmosis
Edited by Judith E. Smith
© Springer-Verlag Berlin Heidelberg 1993

growth have yet been made. In the current paper we report on the early growth and development of *T. gondii* tissue cysts in a robust and efficient model system.

Methods.

<u>Parasites:</u>   Cysts from the ME 49 strain were used to initiate all cultures. Parasite stocks were maintained by intraperitoneal inoculation of adult female outbred mice (Tucks no 1) with approximately 20 cysts harvested from infected brain. For culture, cysts were harvested from infected mouse brain between 1 and 2 months post infection, purified on Percol gradients according to the method of Cornelissen *et al* ., [1981], counted, then disrupted by 35% Pepsin/ HCl for two minutes at room temperature.

In vitro culture: Madin & Darby Bovine Kidney cells were routinely maintained in log phase growth in Ham's F12 medium supplemented with 10% foetal calf serum and 2% Penicillin-Streptomycin-Fungizone (Gibco). For cyst culture $2x10^5$ cells were plated onto 13mm coverslips in Costar multiwell plates (NUNC) and incubated overnight at 37^0C and 5% CO_2. Between 0.5-$1 x 10^4$ bradyzoites were loaded onto each coverslip and left to invade host cells for two hours.   Cultures were then washed to remove extracellular parasites, fresh medium was added at four day intervals during the 14 day culture period.

<u>Microscopy:</u>   Coverslip cultures were fixed and stained in Giemsa at two day intervals to provide a record of cyst growth and development. Periodic Acid Schiff's (PAS) stain was used to differentially visualise bradyzoites; PAS positive amylopectin granules increase in bradyzoites [Dubey & Frenkel 1976]. To assess numbers of nuclei within a cyst a 2% solution of the fluorescent dye Propidium Iodide was dropped onto air dried, formalin fixed cultures. For immunofluoresence coverslips were air dried, acetone fixed and incubated for 30 mins at 37^0C in primary antibody. Cyst specific polyclonal sera (obtained by adsorption of immune mouse sera against tachyzoites), the monoclonal antibody 1F12, which recognises the tachyzoite surface molecule SAG 3 shared by bradyzoites, and control uninfected mouse sera were used as primary antibody. Cultures were then washed in phosphate buffered saline (PBS), incubated in an anti-mouse IgG.FITC conjugate, washed in PBS, mounted in Optifluor and visualised by conventional fluoresence or confocal microscopy.

<u>Assessment of growth:</u>   Cyst number was estimated by counting the total number of cysts on two replicate coverslips, the size and number of nuclei in each cyst was also noted. Single parasites were not scored, in later cultures the distinction between tachyzoites and cysts was made using morphological criteria. The percentage of infected cells was calculated by scoring the number of infected and uninfected cells in 12 fields of view.

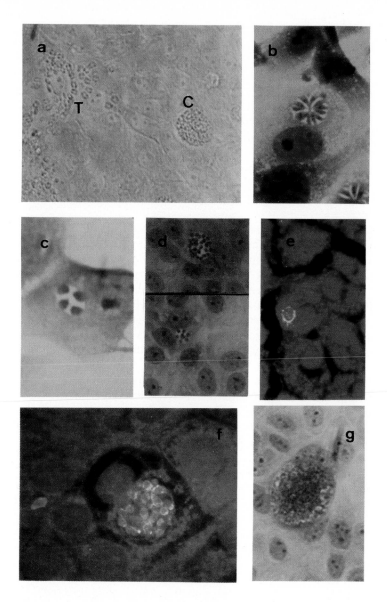

Figure 1. *In vitro* culture of *Toxoplasma gondii* .
Parasites cultured in MDBK cell monolayers a) 10 day bradyzoite initiated
culture containing both cysts (C) and tachyzoites(T): phase contrast. b) typical
rosette structure of dividing tachyzoite in 48hr tachyzoite initiated culture:
giemsa stain. c) 'cruciform' structure' in 48hr bradyzoite initiated culture:
giemsa stain. d) developing cysts with odd numbers of nuclei: giemsa stain. e)
developing cyst visualised with tachyzoite adsorbed polyclonal mouse sera,
exhibiting strong reactivity against the cyst wall: confocal image. f) developing
cyst visualised with monoclonal 1F12 demonstrates SAG 3 on the bradyzoite
surface but not in the cyst wall: confocal image. g) mature cyst in day 12
culture: giemsa stain.

Results.

Development on cysts *in vitro* : morphological data.

In all cultures initiated from bradyzoites the majority of parasites produced cyst like structures and tachyzoites were found only in late cultures (Fig 1a). It was possible to discriminate between these two forms using morphological criteria. Tachyzoite growth is highly synchronous. Following invasion the parasite divides by endodyogeny to form two daughter cells, aligned along their longitudinal axis and contained within a closely opposed parasitophorous vacuole membrane (PV). Subsequent divisions, lead to repeated doubling of the parasite and the formation of rosettes (Fig 1b). Bradyzoite development is different from the very outset.

In the young 'cyst' parasites are rounded or pip shaped, stain positively with PAS and are loosely packed into the PV. During the first divisions parasites are not closely associated and are found around the edge of the vacuole, typically in a 'cruciform' configuration (Fig 1c). Later divisions are asynchronous, and odd numbers of parasites are frequently found within the PV (Fig 1d). Around day 3 to 4 of culture the appearance of the cyst alters, becoming more clearly defined, with parasites contained within a rounded structure, most easily visualised by confocal microscopy. This change is most likely due to assembly of the cyst wall as illustrated via antibody staining. Cyst-specific polyclonal antisera react strongly with this circular wall and rather faintly with the enclosed parasites (Fig 1e), while the monoclonal antibody 1F12, which recognises the shared antigen SAG 3, reacts exclusively with bradyzoites (Fig 1f). Following the formation of the cyst wall parasites continue to divide, however the overall growth rate of the cyst slows and in larger cysts, containing over 100 nuclei, individual bradyzoites appear smaller in size (Fig 1g).

Growth characteristics of *T. gondii* cysts in culture.

The sucessful induction of cysts *in vitro* was estimated by scoring the total number of cysts per coverslip over the fourteen day period of culture. Fig 2 shows the variation in cyst number with time in five replicate experiments, initiated from different batches of bradyzoites. The results are highly reproducible and show little variation between experiments. Cyst number increases rapidly between day 2 and day 6, where numbers reached a peak at 300-500 cysts per coverslip, or approximately 1% of cells infected. After this the total number of cysts started to decline and was still falling at day 14. Over the first four days of culture some cells contained unicellular parasites, however, all dividing parasites had the morphological characteristics of bradyzoites. On day 5-6 of culture tachyzoite like parasites were first seen, these started to amplify in localised areas and multiple infection of host cells was frequently seen (Fig 1a). These tachyzoite like parasites caused focal destruction of the host cell monolayer by day 8-10.

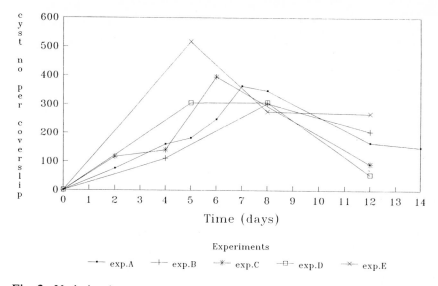

<u>Fig 2.</u> Variation in cyst number per coverslip with time.
The total number of tissue cysts per coverslip, mean of 3 replicates, is plotted for
five replicate experiments using MDBK cells loaded with ME49 strain bradyzoites.

The growth rate of cysts was estimated by calculating the mean diameter of
the population of cysts on each day of culture (Table 1). Over the first few days
of culture the increase in cyst size is rapid and pronounced, but around day 5 growth
slows and the mean cyst size remains constant for the remainder of
the culture period.
The division rate of bradyzoites within the cyst mirrored the increase in cyst
size (Table 1). The mean number of nuclei per cyst showed a rapid early
increase with a mean number of 26 ± 0.9 parasites per cyst on day 6 of culture,
followed by a slower increase to an average of 30 ±1.5 parasites per cyst on
day 14.

<u>Table 1.</u> Growth of *Toxoplasma gondii* tissue cysts: mean diameter and number
of nuclei.

Day of culture	2	4	5	6	7	8	12	14
mean diam	4.6	3.9	7	6.6	7.2	6.1	6	6.6
μm	±0.2	±0.3	±0.2	±0.1	±0.1	±0.4	±0.2	±0.7
mean no	12.1	10.7	20.8	26.2	28.2	25.4	22.1	30.5
nuclei	±0.3	±0.8	±1.6	±1.0	±0.9	±0.9	±1.4	±1.5

Data are based on total counts of all cysts on replicate coverslips (n≤100)

Overall it can be seen that a cohort of cysts was produced from bradyzoite initiated cultures and that growth and maturation of these cysts is well synchronised over the first 4-6 days of culture. In later cultures the growth rate of cysts apparently slows. Frequency analysis of nuclear number data, showed that by day 8 of culture, two populations of cysts were emerging: small (3-30 nuclei), and large (40+ nuclei). By day 12 of culture the majority of cysts were small, but some were very large with over 150 nuclei. This implies that there is some turnover of cysts but that a subset of the first cohort of cysts matures fully over the 14 day period of culture.

Bradyzoite:tachyzoite conversion.

In the current series of experiments parasites exhibiting typical tachyzoite growth were first seen after 6 days of culture, but the division rate of these parasites was high and by 14 days over 4% of cells were infected and damage to the monolayer was apparent. This pattern of bradyzoite:tachyzoite conversion was noted in cultures initiated with several strains of *T. gondii* (ME49, Beverley, 18692, 17025). Further, serial passage of parasites obtained during culture always resulted in mixed tachyzoite, bradyzoite cultures. In contrast cultures initiated from tachyzoites of the virulent RH and Martin strains normally resulted in total monolayer destruction by tachyzoites, however in larger scale culture (25cm^2 flasks) cysts were occasionally seen .

Discussion.

Studies of tissue cysts *in vivo* reveal several features associated with this stage. The cyst, contained within its thick fibrillar wall is believed to have a very slow metabolic rate and a long lifespan. Indeed it was originally suggested that cysts survived for the lifespan of the host, although more recently evidence of cyst turnover [Frenkel & Escajadillo 1987, Ferguson *et al* ., 1989] and of turnover of bradyzoites within the cyst [Pavesio *et al* ., 1992] has come to light. Cysts are found in a subset of cells in brain and muscle tissue, giving rise to the suggestion that host cell metabolism might induce tachyzoite:bradyzoite conversion and cyst growth. Finally it has been suggested that cyst formation and stability is essentially under immunological control. Certainly the appearance of cysts coincides with the onset of immunity and it has been suggested that specific immunomodulators, such as γ−IFN, prevent cyst rupture and recrudesence of the disease [Suzuki *et al* ., 1989].

Direct evaluation of tachyzoite:bradyzoite conversion rates, cyst growth, survival and turnover can only be made *in vitro* . A limited number of these studies have attempted to mimic conditions found *in vivo*, for example, Shimada *et al*., [1974] related production of tissue cysts, from RH strain tachyzoites in rabbit corneal endothelium, to the presence of high titres of immune serum and complement. Jones *et al* ., [1986] cultured Pe strain bradyzoites in primary cultures of mouse astrocytes, they reinforced findings that γ-IFN inhibits tachyzoite growth [Pfefferkorn 1984] and further suggested that it prevented cyst rupture.

The majority of reports, however, suggest the production of cysts is not dependent on host cell type, culture medium or presence of immunological factors [Hogan et al ., 1960, Hoff et al ., 1977, Lindsay et al ., 1991, Darde et al ., 1989]. In the current experiment we have used a culture system originally designed for studies of tachyzoite invasion and growth [Grimwood & Smith 1992], as the host cell type and culture conditions are identical any difference in growth and development must be directed solely by the parasite.

Our morphological observations of bradyzoites in culture suggest that from the outset the relationship with the host cell is different to that of the tachyzoite. The parasites are loosely contained within a relatively large parasitophorous vacuole and, perhaps most interesting, the cell cycle of the dividing zoites is no longer synchronous, so that rather than the usual tachyzoite 2, 4, 8, 16 configuration we see a high frequency of odd numbers within the young cyst.

It is quite conceivable that adaptation of the parasitophorous membrane is different with bradyzoites and that this may influence development of the cyst. Certainly this stage does not possess the major surface antigen SAG 1, believed to act as a ligand in tachyzoite invasion [Grimwood & Smith 1992, Kasper this volume]. In fact the bradyzoite surface shares only two antigens with the tachyzoite (SAG 3 & 4) and bears at least four stage specific molecules (BAG 1-4) [Tomavo et al 1991, Soete this volume]. The role of these molecules, and indeed of those in rhoptries and dense granules, in invasion and PV formation remains to be determined.

Early cyst development occurs very rapidly and after three days in culture formation of the cyst wall is in progress. The nature of this wall is again poorly understood, direct labelling studies [Woodison 1992] suggest that it is enriched in bradyzoite molecules including two of Mr 21,000 and 34,000 (' BAG 1 & 3'). The formation of the wall is a critical event in cyst maturation. Its thick fibrillar structure [Ferguson & Hutchinson 1987] must alter the traffic of molecules between parasite and host cell and will certainly prevent any membrane associated transfer. In culture, cyst rupture is most frequent between days 3 and 6, but those cysts which survive this phase carry on to produce mature cysts by day 10-14.

One major aim in developing the culture system was to study the relationship between bradyzoites and tachyzoites and the developmental programme which controls switching between these two stages. In common with other authors [Shimada et al ., 1974, Jones et al ., 1986, Lindsay et al ., 1992] we have found that cultures initiated with tachyzoites of the virulent RH and Martin strains will produce more tachyzoites and the frequency of switching to bradyzoite is minimal, while in cultures initiated from newly released bradyzoites of 'avirulent' strains very few tachyzoites are found initially and there is a low rate of switching to the tachyzoite form. We propose that the rate of switching between the two stages is intrinsic to the parasite, that in virulent parasites the rate of T>B (tachyzoite to bradyzoite) switching is very much lower than the B>T rate, while in avirulent strains a closer balance is set.

Logically the switch which controls differentiation is likely to act on each individual parasite at a point prior to cell division. It is important to determine firstly, whether these intrinic rates of switching exist and secondly, if the switch is also sensitive to environmental cues (eg PV derived from bradyzoite or tachyzoite; parasite within existing mature cyst; high γ-IFN levels). This can be achieved by using stage specific marker molecules to identify tachyzoites and bradyzoites in culture. Recently Dubremetz and co-workers demonstrated that two populations of parasites bearing tachyzoite, or the bradyzoite specific marker molecules, can coexist in the same vacuole [Soete et al ., this volume]. This does imply that control operates at the level of individual parasites and it is therefore important to extend these studies to gain numerical data on conversion rates.

In summary we have developed a robust culture system which allows us to follow the synchronous development of a cohort of cysts. The efficiency of the system is remarkable, a single coverslip will yield up to 500 cysts, this compares favourably with numbers harvested from mouse brain (approx 1,500). The system will enable metabolic studies of early cyst development and cell wall assembly, cellular investigations of bradyzoite invasion and parasitophorous vacuole formation and bradyzoite turnover in the cyst. Moreover, with the use of appropriate antibody probes,we may be able to determine the kinetics of bradyzoite:tachyzoite conversion and thus gain insight into differentiation.

Acknowledgements. This work was supported by a grant from the Agriculture and Food Research Council. We are indebted to Ms Debra Evans for technical assistance.

References.

Achbarou, A., Mercereau-Puijalon, O., Autheman, J.M., Fortier, B., Camus, C., Dubremetz, J.F [1991] Characterization of microneme proteins of T oxoplasma gondii. Mol. Biochem. Parasitol. 47: 223-234.

Burg, J.L., Perleman, D., Kasper, L.L., Ware, P.L., Boothroyd, J.C. [1988] Molecular analysis of the gene encoding the major surface antigen of Toxoplasma gondii. J. Immunol.141: 3584-3591.

Cesbron-Delauw, M.F., Guy, B., Torpier, G., Pierce, R.J., Lenzen, G., Cesbron, J.Y., Charif, H., Lepage, P., Darcy, F., Lecocq, J.P., Capron, A. [1989] Molecular characterization of a 23-KDa major antigen secreted by Toxoplasma gondii. Proc. Natl. Acad. Sci. USA. 86: 7537-7541.

Coernelissen, A.W.C.A., Overdulve, J.P., Hoenderboom, J.M. [1981] Separation of Isospora (Toxoplasma) gondii cysts and cystozoites from mouse brain by continuous density gradient centrifugation. J. Parasitol. 83: 103-108.

Couvreur, G., Sadak, A., Fortier, B,. Dubremetz, J.F. [1988] Surface antigens of Toxoplasma gondii.. Parasitol. 97: 1-10.

Darde, M.L., Bouteille, B., Leboutet, M.J., Loubet, A., Pestre-Alexandre, M. [1989] *Toxoplasma gondii* : etude ultrastructurale des formations kistiques observees en culture de fibroblastes humains. Ann. Parasitol. Hum. Comp. 64: 403-411

Dubey, J.P., Frenkel, J.K. [1976] Feline toxoplasmosis from acutely infected mice and the development of *Toxoplasma* cysts. J. Protozool. 23: 537-546.

Ferguson, D.J.P., Hutchinson, W.M. [1987] An ultrastructural study of the early development and tissue cyst formation of *Toxoplasma gondii* in the brains of mice. Parasitol. Res. 73: 483-491.

Ferguson, D.J.P., Hutchinson, W.M., Petterson, E. [1989] Tissue cyst rupture in mice chronically infected with *Toxoplasma gondii* : an immuno-cytochemical and ultrastructural study. Parasitol. Res. 75: 599-603.

Frenkel, J.K., Escajadillo, A. [1987] Cyst rupture as a pathogenic mechanism of toxoplasmic encephalitis. Am. J.Trop. Med. Hyg. 36: 517-522.

Grimwood, J., Smith, J.E. [1992] *Toxoplasma gondii* : The role of a 30-kDa surface protein in host cell invasion. Exp. Parasitol. 74: 106-111.

Hoff, R.L., Dubey, J.P., Behbehani, A.M., Frenkel, J.K. [1977] *Toxoplasma gondii* cysts in cell culture: new biologic evidence. J. Parasitol. 63: 1121-1124.

Hogan, M.J., Yoneda, C., Feeney, L., Zweigart, P., Lewis, A. [1960] Morphology and culture of *Toxoplasma* . Arch. Opthal. 64: 655-667.

Jones, T.C., Bienz, K.A., Erb, P. [1986] *In vitro* cultivation of *Toxoplasma gondii* cysts in astrocytes in the presence of gamma interferon. Infect. Immun. 51: 146-156.

Kasper, L.H., Crabb, J.H., Pfefferkorn, E. [1983] Purification of a major membrane protein of *Toxoplasma gondii* by immunoabsorbtion with a monoclonal antibody. J. Immunol. 130: 2407-2412.

Kasper, L.H. [1989] Identification of stage-specific antigens of *Toxoplasma gondii* . Infect.Immun. 57: 668-672.

Leriche, M.A., Dubremetz, J.F. [1991] Characterisation of the proteins of rhoptries and dense granules of *Toxoplasma gondii* by subcellular fractionation and monoclonal antibodies. Mol. Biochem. Parasitol .45: 249-260.

Lindsay, D.S., Dubey, J.P., Blagburn, B.L., Toivio-Kinnucan, M. [1991] Examination of tissue cyst formation by *Toxoplasma gondii* in cell cultures using bradyzoites, tachyzoites, and sporozoites. J. Parasitol. 77:126-132

Luft, B.J., Remington, J.S. [1988] AIDS commentary: Toxoplasmic encephalitis. J. Infect. Dis. 157: 1-6.

Omata, Y., Igarshi, M., Ramos, M.I., Nakabayashi, T. [1989] *Toxoplasma gondii* : Antigenic differences between endozoites and cystozoites defined with monoclonal antibodies. Parasitol. Res. 75: 189-193.

Ossorio, P.N., Schwartzman, J.D., Boothroyd, J.C. [1992] A *Toxoplasma gondii* rhoptry protein associated with invasion has unusual charge asymmetry. Mol. Bioch. Parasit. 50: 1-16.

Pavesio, C.E.N., Chiappino, M.L., Setzer, P.Y., Nichols, B.A. [1992] *Toxoplasma gondii* : differentiation and death of bradyzoites. Parasitol. Res. 78: 1-9.

Pfefferkorn, E.R. [1984] Interferon-γ blocks the growth of *Toxoplasma gondii* in human fibroblasts by inducing the host cells to degrade tryptophan. Proc. Natl. Acad. Sci. USA 81: 908-912.

Shimada, K., O' Connor, R., Yoneda, C. [1974] Cyst formation by *Toxoplasma gondii* (RH strain) in vitro. Arch. Opthalmol. 92: 496-500

Suzuki, Y., Conley, F.K., Remington, J.S. [1989] Importance of endogenous γ-IFN for prevention of toxoplasmic encephalitis in mice. J. Immunol. 143: 2045-2050.

Tomavo, S., Fortier, B., Soerte, M., Ansel, C., Camus, D., Dubremetz, J-F. [1991] Characterization of bradyzoite specific antigens of *Toxoplasma gondii* . Infect. Immun. 59: 3750-3753.

Weiss, L.M., Laplace, D., Tanowitz, H.B., Whittner, M. [1992] Identification of *Toxoplasma gondii* bradyzoite specific monoclonal antibodies. J. Infect. Dis. 166: 4350-4354.

Woodison, G. [1992] *Toxoplasma gondii* : antigenic overlap between tachyzoites and tissue cysts. PhD Thesis, University of Leeds.

Woodison, G., Smith, J.E., [1990] Identification of the dominant cyst antigens of *Toxoplasma gondii* . Parasitol. 100: 389-392.

Zhang, Y.W., Smith, J.E. *Toxoplasma gondii*: Identification and characterisation of a cyst specific antigen. submitted.

RECENT ADVANCES IN THE GLYCOBIOLOGY OF *TOXOPLASMA GONDII*

Ralph T. Schwarz, Stanislas Tomavo*, Maria Odenthal-Schnittler, Boris Striepen, Dirk Becker, Martina Eppinger, Christina F. Zinecker and Jean François Dubremetz**

Zentrum für Hygiene und Medizinische Mikrobiologie,
Philipps-Universität Marburg,
W-3550 Marburg,
Germany

Posttranslational modifications of proteins by oligossaccharides and glycolipids play an important role for the structure, biosynthesis and biological function of surface membrane proteins of viruses, bacteria and eukaryotic cells including parasitic protozoa. Until recently very little on the glycobiology of *Toxoplasma gondii* was known and considerable controversy as to the presence of glycoproteins as major surface components of the Toxoplasma existed [Handman et al., 1980; Johnson et al., 1981; Mauras et al., 1980; Naot et al., 1983; Sharma et al., 1983]. It has now become apparent that the major membrane surface proteins of T. gondii are modified by glycoconjugates. Their role in the biology and pathology of the parasite remains to be elucidated in detail.

Introduction

The dolichol-cycle of protein N-glycosylation

The glycosylation of proteins containing oligosaccharides N-linked to asparagine proceeds in two stages. Firstly, the precursor oligosaccharide Glc3Man9(GlcNAc)2 is assembled on a dolichol pyrophosphate carrier in the rough endoplasmic reticulum. In the second stage, following its transfer to the nascent polypeptide, the precursor oligosaccharide undergoes a series of processing reactions in the rough endoplasmic reticulum and in the Golgi apparatus, resulting in the formation of the high-mannosidic and complex-type oligosaccharides, characteristic of mature asparagine-linked glycoproteins. It is possible to manipulate both, the formation of the lipid-linked oligosaccharide precursor in the Dolichol cycle and the oligosaccharide processing by specific inhibitors. For reviews see Kornfeld and Kornfeld, 1985; McDowell and Schwarz, 1988; Elbein, 1987.

---

* Dept. of Microbiology and Immunology, Stanford Univ. School of Medicine, Fairchild Bldg. D305, Stanford, CA 94305-5402, USA
** Unité 42 de l'INSERM, 369 rue Jules Guesde, 59650 Villeneuve d'Ascq, France

NATO ASI Series, Vol. H 78
Toxoplasmosis
Edited by Judith E. Smith
© Springer-Verlag Berlin Heidelberg 1993

O-glycosylation

Another type of glycosylation is the attachment of carbohydrate chains to selected serine and/or threonine residues. In contrast to N-glycosylation the carbohydrate residues are attached to the proteins in a stepwise manner leading to a variety of glycans. The linkage between serine or threonine and the first sugar is labile against the exposure to "mild alkali" (e. g. 0.1 N NaOH, 16 hrs, 45oC, 0.5 - 2.0 M NaBH4) leading to a fragmentation reaction known as ß-elimination [Sharon, 1975] which is diagnostic for O-linked carbohydrates in proteins.

Although the participation of a lipid-linked sugar, Dol-P-Man, has been described to play a role in the formation of the serine-bound and threonine bound oligomannose chains in the yeast *Saccharomyces cerevisiae* [Sharma et al., 1974; Lehle and Tanner, 1975] sugar nucleotides are the principal donors acting in concert in the Golgi apparatus which is the main site of O-glycan formation.

Glycosylphosphatidylinositol membrane anchors

A recently detected class of proteins are attached to eukaryotic cell surfaces via inositol-containing glycophospholipids (GPIs). The glycolipid anchors are first synthesized as precursor glycolipids which are then covalently linked to target proteins in the endoplasmic reticulum (ER). In all reported cases, the lipid anchor replaces a short sequence of mainly hydrophobic amino acids at the carboxy terminus of the protein [cf. Ferguson and Williams, 1988]. Most of the information on the structure and biosynthesis of glycolipid membrane anchors has been obtained from studies of the variant surface glycoproteins (VSGs) and GPIs of the parasitic protozoan, *Trypanosoma brucei*. The glycolipid anchor of one VSG (VSG 117) has been completely chemically defined and consists of the backbone sequence ethanolamine-phosphate-6Mana1-2Mana1-6Mana1-4GlcNa1-6inositol. The inositol residue is linked via a phosphodiester bond to dimyristoylglycerol, the ethanolamine group is amide-linked to the carboxy terminal amino acid of the mature protein and a galactose side-chain is attached to the mannose residue adjacent to glucosamine. Similar backbone structures with different side-chain modifications and lipophilic groups have been described for the lipid anchors of some other proteins [for reviews see Ferguson and Williams, 1988; Cross 1990].

Two candidate glycolipid precursors have been identified in *Trypanosoma brucei* [Menon et al., 1988; Krakow et al., 1986]. They are GPI species containing a single N-unsubstituted ethanolamine residue, a Man3GlcN core glycan identical to the backbone sequence of the VSG glycolipid anchor, and a dimyristoyl-phosphatidylinositol moiety. One, P2 (lipid A), like the VSG glycolipid anchor, is cleaved by phosphatidylinositol specific phospholipase C (PI-PLC). The second, P3 (lipid C), is insusceptible to this enzyme due to a fatty acid esterified to the inositol ring.

The glycolipid precursors P2 (lipid A) and P3 (lipid C) along with their putative biosynthetic intermediates have been synthesized in cell free systems [Menon et al., 1990a; Masterson et al., 1989] by incubating radiolabeled sugar nucleotides with crude preparations of trypanosome membranes. Structural analysis of the resulting labeled lipids suggest that GPI species are most probably assembled by sequential addition of monosaccharides to phosphatidyl-inositol (PI). Assembly begins with the transfer of GlcNAc via UDP-GlcNAc to PI. Subsequent deacetylation of GlcNAc-PI gives GlcN-PI. The glycolipid then appears to be built up by the stepwise addition of three mannose residues and the terminal ethanolamine phosphate group.

Work from several laboratories suggests that one or more of the mannose residues in the GPI glycan is derived from a lipid-linked mannose donor, dolichol-P-mannose. Further evidence is derived from experiments with 2-fluoro-2-deoxy-glucose and Amphomycin, two inhibitors of dolichol-P-mannose synthesis, that all three mannose residues in the GPI glycan are derived from dolichol-P-mannose [Schwarz et al., 1989; Menon et al., 1990; for a review see Cross, 1990]. The lipid moiety of the trypanosomal GPI-membrane anchor undergoes extensive "remodelling" resulting in the replacement by myristic acid of the acyl groups bound to glycerol [Masterson et al., 1990; cf. Doering et al, 1990].

The Glycosylphosphatidylinositols of *T. gondii*

The major surface proteins of *T. gondii* are anchored to the parasites surface by a GPI-membrane anchor [Tomavo et al., 1989; Nagel et al., 1989]. In addition an immunogenic lipophilic component [Sharma et al., 1983] detectable early after infections and migrating to the front of an SDS gel was characterized in some detail.

Glycosylphosphatidylinositols assumed to be candidate precursors of toxoplasmal glycosylphosphatidyl membrane anchors.

T. gondii tachyzoites, RH strain, grown in cultures of Vero cells were incubated with radiolabeled precursors known to be components of GPI-membrane anchors. At the end of the labeling period, parasites were washed with phosphate buffered saline and extracted with chloroform/methanol (CM, 2:1) to remove neutral lipids, phospholipids and less polar glycolipids. The CM-residual pellet was then extracted with chloroform/methanol/water (CMW, 10:10:3) to obtain more polar glycolipids. The CMW-extracted glycolipids were partitioned between water and water-saturated n-butanol. Analysis and purification of CM-extractable glycolipids and of the `butanol component´ of the CMW extract was done by thin layer chromatography.

The obtained lipid fractions were analyzed by specific enzymatic and/or chemical treatments followed by analysis on thin layer chromatography, Biogel P4, or High pH exchange chromatography, HPAEC (BioLC-HPLC apparatus, Dionex Corp., CA). Four major glycolipids from *Toxoplasma gondii* tachyzoites were found in the 'butanol component' of the CMW extracts which were metabolically labelled with tritiated glucosamine, mannose, palmitic- and myristic acid, ethanolamine, and inositol. They were designated A, B, C and D. Glycolipids A, B, and C contain at least one ethanolaminephosphate residue. Judging from their sensitivity to a set of enzymatic tests and chemical fragmentation reactions, the glycoplipids A, B and C share several properties with the glycoplipid moiety of the GPI anchor of the major surface proteins P30 and P23 of *T. gondii*. They contain a nonacetylated glucosamine-inositol phosphate-linkage (which is diagnostic for GPIs), they are sensitive toward phosphatidylinositol-specific phospholipase C and nitrous acid treatment and show identical glycan backbones as judged by HPAEC after HF-dephosphorylation. All are characterized by the presence of a linear core glycan structure ending with an ethanolamine phosphate residue. Taken together with the nature of radiolabelled precursors incorporated into these glycolipids, the data indicates that these GPIs are involved in the biosynthesis of the GPI-membrane anchors of *T. gondii* and may represent different degrees of completion [Tomavo et al., 1992a].

The dephosphorylated glycans from glycoplids A, B, and C are identical to the dephosphorylated glycans of the GPI anchors of P23 and P30, whereas glycolipid D is different from the other glycolipids in its glycan backbone. Its role is unknown and remains to be elucidated.

Although labelling of cultures of *T. gondii* proved to be helpful in identifying GPIs of *T. gondii* it was desirable to establish a cell-free system to study their synthesis in detail allowing the manipulation of more parameters than under *in vivo* conditions.

Incubation of membranes prepared using a modification of the method described by Masterson et al. [1989] with radioactive sugar nucleotides (GDP-[^{3}H]Mannose or UDP-[^{3}H]GlcNAc) resulted in incorporation of radiolabel into numerous glycoplipids. Using a combination of chemical/enzymatic tests followed by chromatographic analysis, a series of incompletely glycosylated lipid species and mature GPIs have been identified. Four glycolipids were detected in the 'butanol component' of the CMW extracts shown to be glycolipids B and D (previously found in culture) and their lyso species designated B' and D' not observed *in vivo*. This may suggest that fatty acid remodelling, which was described in the African trypanosome [Masterson et al., 1990] also occurs in *T. gondii* but does not go to completion *in vitro* resulting in the accumulation of lyso-intermediates. We have also established the involvement of Dol-P-mannose in the synthesis of *T. gondii* GPIs. Altogether our data suggest that the GPI-core glycan in *T. gondii* is assembled via sequential glycosylation of phosphatidyl-inositol, as proposed for the biosynthesis of GPIs in

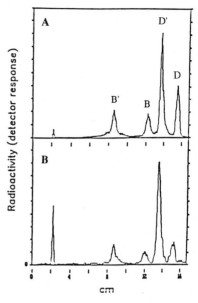

Fig.1 Thin layer chromatography of CMW-extractable glycolipids labeled in the cell-free system via GDP-[^{3}H]Mannose (A) or UDP-[^{3}H]GalNAc (B).

Trypanosoma brucei [Tomavo et al., 1992b; Tomavo et al., 1992c].

In contrast to all free GPIs identified in *T. brucei* and mammalian cells so far, *T. gondii* mature GPI-precursors contain an N-acetylgalactosamine (GalNAc) residue linked to the conserved GPI-core glyan. The observation that UDP-[^{3}H]GalNAc efficiently labels GPIs in the cell-free system (Fig. 1) makes *T. gondii* an interesting model to study in detail the transfer of GalNAc to GPIs and the donors involved. A summary of GPI biosynthesis in *T. gondii* is shown in Fig. 2.

The lipophilic "low molecular weight (LMW)" antigen

Using human patient sera, previous studies have described a lipophilic low molecular weight ("LMW") antigen, which elicits an IgM response in human primary infection [Sharma et al., 1993]. Monoclonal antibodies specific for this antigen have recently been obtained [Tomavo et al., 1992d], and were used to characterize the "LMW" antigen.

RH-strain tachyzoites were propagated in cultures of Vero cells. Metabolically labelled or unlabelled parasites were released from the cells and extracted with CM followed by two extractions with CMW. CMW-extractable molecules were subjected to SDS-PAGE followed by transfer to nitrocellulose sheets and characterization by two monoclonal antibodies (T54E10 and T33F12) and sera from humans with an acute toxoplasmosis (kindly provided by Dr B Fortier, CHU Lille). It could be demonstrated by enzymatic and chemical reactions in conjunction with metabolic labelling that the low molecular weight antigen of *Toxoplasma gondii* is a family of glycosyl-inositolphospholips [Striepen, 1991; Striepen et al., 1992].

Work is underway to compare the GPIs of the "low molecular weight antigen" with the GPIs assumed to be condidates for toxoplasmal GPI-membrane anchors.

Fig. 2 Hypothetical scheme of the biosynthetic pathways for *T. gondii* GPIs in the cell-free system.

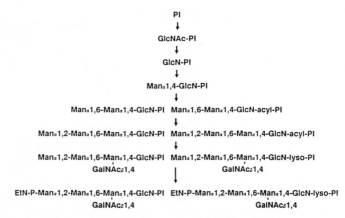

Characterization of toxoplasmal GPI-membrane anchors

It is of fundamental importance to compare protein-bound GPIs with their putative precursor molecules in order to establish a detailed biosynthetic pathway. Therefore the GPI-membrane anchors of the major surface glycoproteins P23 and P30 were analyzed in some detail. P23 was metabolically labelled with tritiated palmitate, myristate, ethanolamine, inositol, glucosamine, and mannose, known to be components of GPI-anchor structures.

P23 was released from the surface of living parasites by treatment with phosphatidylinositol-specific phospholipase C (PI-PLC) and the resulting water-soluble protein was immunoprecipitated with a monoclonal antibody specific for P23. The GPI-core glycan was generated after aqueous-HF dephosphorylation followed by nitrous deamination and its carbohydrate structure was characterized using selective exo- and endoglycosidase treatments. Finally, the phosphatidylinositol moiety of P23 was characterized using PI-PLC and phospholipase A_2 digestions. Our cumulative data P23 of *T. gondii* tachyzoites contains the highly conserved backbone, consisting of ethanolamine-P-6Manα1-2Manα1-6Manα1-4GlcNα1-6PI with a side-chain modification which was identified as a N-acetylgalactosamine residue, similar to the mammalian Thy-1 anchor [cf. Ferguson et al., 1988; Tomavo et al, 1992e].

A comparable analysis was undertaken for P30 with analogous results [Tomavo et al., 992a; Zinecker et al., 1992]. Thus, the anchors of both proteins are identical with respect to their carbohydrate moieties. Some microheterogeneity for the glycan of P30 has been demonstrated [Zinecker, 1992] and it remains to be investigated if this is a common feature of toxoplasmal GPI-membrane anchors

Evidence for N- and O-glycosylation of toxoplasmal proteins

Evidence for N-glycosylation of P23
It was of particular interest to investigate whether *T. gondii* is able to perform N-glycosylation as it was recently described that the dolichol cycle of N-glycosylation appears to be absent in asexual erythrocytic stages of *Plasmodium falciparum*, another apicomplexan protozoan [Dieckmann-Schuppert et al., 1992]. Inhibitors of glycosylation or trimming (diagnostic for N-glycosylation) such as 2-deoxy-D-glucose, 2-deoxy-2-fluoro-D-glucose, 2-deoxy-2-fluoro-D-mannose, tunicamycin or N-methyl-deoxynojirimycin [Schwarz and Datema, 1982; Schwarz and Datema, 1984; Elbein, 1987] did not interfere with the multiplication of *Toxoplasma gondii* up to a concentration of 10 mM [Dubremetz and Schwarz, unpublished observation). Thus, as the membrane of the parasitophorous vacuole might, under the applied experimental conditions, represent a protecting barrier against the tested compounds the question of whether *T. gondii* is capable of N-glycosylation was directly approached.

P23 labelled with [³H]-glucosamine was purified from detergent solubilized material using monoclonal antibodies coupled to sepharose 4B-CNBr. The resulting glycopeptides of pronase digested proteins cut out of a SDS-gel were sized by gel-permeation chromatography on Biogel P4. Four peaks with V_e/V_o- values of 1.41, 1.45, 1.53 and 1.61 were identified which shift to positions corresponding to V_e/V_o values of 1.49, 1.56, 1.64, and 1.74 after incubation with PNGase F, an enzyme known to specifically release N-glycans from proteins (Fig. 3). Further proof for N-glycosylation in *T. gondii* is derived from supplementary biochemical studies. A cell-free system was

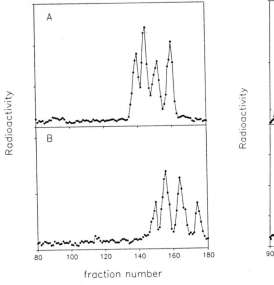

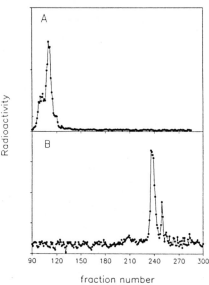

Fig.3 Chromatography of glycopeptides derived from pronase digests of [³H]-glucosamine-labeled P23 prior (A) and after treatment with PNGase F.

Fig.4 Chromatography of glycopeptides derived from pronase digests of [³H]-glucosamine-labeled P28 prior (A) and after ß-elimination.

established from isolated tachyzoites which is capable of synthesizing at least one of the precursors known to be involved in N-glycosylation of eukaryotic cells, namely $Man_9(GlcNAc)_2$-PP-Dol. Further studies are needed to resolve the question whether higher, glucosylated species are also formed and whether they are transferred to toxoplasmal proteins and subsequently trimmed. The capability of *T. gondii* tachyzoites to synthesize $Man_9(GlcNAc)_2$-PP-Dol

[Odenthal-Schnittler et al., 1992, Odenthal-Schnittler et al., 1993] suggests that *T. gondii* has its own glycosylating machinery to N-glycosylate toxoplasmal proteins.

Preliminary studies concerning the O-glycosylation of toxoplasmal protein

P28 is a protein found in dense granules [Charif et al., 1990; Sibley and Sharma, 1987] and it has been reported that it was strongly labelled with [^{3}H]-glucosamine [Archbarou et al., 1991]. P28 labelled with [^{3}H]-glucosamine was purified from detergent solublized material using monoclonal antibodies coupled to sepharose 4B-CNBr. The resulting glycopeptides of pronase digested proteins cut out of a SDS-gel were sized by gel-permeation chromatography on Biogel P4. A broad peak eluting with V_o was found to be insensitive to PNGase F, endo F, and endo H, enzymes known to act on N-glycans. After β-elimination (0.1 N NaOH, 16 hrs, 45°C, 0.5 M NaBH$_4$) however, two peaks were found with V_e/V_o values of 2.53 and 2.62 [Fig. 4; Odenthal-Schnittler et al., 1992]. Preliminary data obtained by the use of exoglycosidases suggests that they may represent O-linked GalNAc-Gal and GalNAc [Odenthal-Schnittler, Tomavo and Schwarz, unpublished observation] occurring in a cluster of a serine/threonine rich segment of the amino acid sequence resulting in large glycopeptides containing serveral O-linked glycans which would account for the elution property of the untreated glycopeptide.

Future studies

It will be important to elucidate in detail the structures of the GPI-membrane anchors with respect to their glycan and lipid moieties and of the N- and O-linked glycans and to search for structural features not found in mammalian cells.

In addition we will focus on the pathways involved to learn more about the glycobiology of *T. gondii*.

Conclusion

Advances have been made towards an undertstanding of the glycobiology of *T. gondii* tachyzoites. In addition to N- and O-glycans *T. gondii* tachyzoites synthesize GPIs which anchor membrane proteins to the plasma membrane and may play a role in the immunology and diagnosis of toxoplasmosis. Parasite-specific glycoconjugate structures may become targets for specific inhibitors to be developed in the future.

Acknowledgements

This work was supported by SFB 286 from he Deutsche Forschungsgemeinschaft (FG), Fonds der Chemischen Industrie, Stiftung P.E. Kempkes, PROCOPE from ANRT/DAAD, Hessisches Ministerium für Wissenschaft und Kunst, Institut National de la Sante et de la Recherche Medicale (I.N.S.E.R.M) and Centre National de al Recherche Scientifique (C.N.R.S.).
B.S. thanks the Friedrich Ebert Foundation for a scholarship and S.T. is indebted to the Alexander von Humboldt Foundation for a post-doctoral fellowship. C.F.Z. thanks the Hessische Graduiertenforderung for a scholarship.

References

Achbarou, A., Mercerau-Puijalon, O., Sadak, A., Fortier, B., Leriche, M.A., Camus, D., and Dubremetz, J.F. [1991]. Differential targeting of dense granule proteins in the parasitophorous vacuole of *Toxoplasma gondii*. Parasitol 103, 321-329.

Charif, H., Darcy, F., Torpier, G., Cesbron-Delauw, M.F., and Capron, A. [1990]. *Toxoplasma gondii:* Characterization and localization of antigens secreted from tachyzoites. Exp Parasitol 71, 114-124.

Cross, G.A.M. [1990]. Glycolipid anchoring of plasma membrane proteins. Annu. Rev. Cell Biol. 6, 1-39.

Dieckmann-Schuppert, A., Bender, S., Odenthal-Schnittler, M., Bause, E., and Schwarz, R.T. [1992]. Apparent lack of N-glycosylation in the asexual intraerythrocytic stage of *Plasmodium falciparum*. Eur. J. Biochem. 205 (2) 815-825.

Doering, T.L., Masterson, W.J., Hart, G.W., and Englund, P.T. [1990]. Biosynthesis of glycosylphosphatidyl inositol membrane anchors. J. Biochem. 265, 611-614.

Elbein, A.D. [1987]. Inhibitors of the biosynthesis and processing of N-linked oligosaccharde chains. Annu. Rev. Biochem. 56, 497-534.

Ferguson, M.A.J. and Williams, A.F. [1988]. Cell-surface anchoring proteins via glycosyl-phosphatidylinositol structures. Ann. Rev. Biochem. 57, 285-320.

Handman, E., Goding, J.W., and Remington, J.S. [1980]. Detection and characterization of membrane antigens of *Toxoplasma gondii*. J. Immunol. 124, 2578-2583.

Johnson, A.M., McDonald, P.J., and Neoh, S.H. [1981]. Molecular weight anlysis of the major polypeptides and glycopeptides of *Toxoplasma gondii*. Biochem. Biophys. Res. Commun. 100, 934-943.

Kornfeld, R. and Kornfeld, S. [1985]. Assembly of asparagine-lined oligosacchardies. Annu. Rev. Biochem. 54, 631-664.

Krakow, J.L., Hereld, D., Bangs, J.D., Hart, G.W., and Englund, P.T. [1986]. Identification of a glycolipid precursor of the *Trypanosoma brucei* variant surface glycoprotein. J. Biol. Chem. 261, 12147-12153.

Lehle, L. and Tanner, W. [1975]. Formation of lipid-bound oligosaccharides in yeast. Biochim. Biophys. Acta, 399, 364-374.

Masterson, W.J., Doehring, T.L., Hart, G.W., and Englund, P.T. [1989]. A novel pathway for glycan assembly: biosynthesis of the glycosyl-phosphatidylinositol anchor of the trypanosome variant surface glycoprotein. Cell. 56, 793-800.

Masterson, W.J., Raper, J., Doering, T.L., Hart, G.W., and Englund, P.T. [1990]. Fatty acid remodeling: a novel reaction sequence in the biosynthesis of trypanosome glycosyl phosphatidylinositol membrane anchors. Cell. 62, 73-80.

Mauras, G., Dodeur, M., Laget, P. Senet, J.M., and Bourillon, R., [1980]. Partial resolution of the sugar content of *Toxoplasma gondii* membrane. Biochim. Biophys. Res. Commun. 97, 906-912.

McDowell, W., and Schwarz, R.T. [1988]. Dissecting glycoprotein biosynthesis by use of specific inhibitors. Biochimie. 70, 1535-1549.

Menon, A.K., Mayor, S., Ferguson, M.A.J., Duszenko, M., and Cross, G.A.M. [1988]. Candidate glycophospholipid precursor for the glycosylphosphatidylinositol membrane anchor of *Trypanosoma brucei* variant surface glycoproteins. J. Biol. Chem. 263, 1970-1977.

Menon, A.K., Schwarz, R.T., Mayor, S., and Cross, G.A.M. [1990a] Cell-free synthesis of glycosylphosphatidylinositol precursors for the glycoplipid membrane anchor of *Trypanosoma brucei* variant surface glycoproteins. J. Biol. Chem. 265, 9033-9042.

Menon, A.K., Mayor, S., and Schwrz, R.T. [1990b]. Biosynthesis of glycosyl-phosphatidylinositol lipids: involvement of mannosylphosphoryl dolichol. EMBO J. 9, 4249-4258.

Nagel, S.D. and Boothroyd, J.C. [1989]. The major surface antigen, P30, of *Toxoplasma gondii* is anchored by a glycoplipid. J. Biol. Chem. 264, 5569-5574.

Naot, Y., Guptill, D., Mullenax, J., and Remington, J.S. [1983]. Characterisation of *Toxoplasma gondii* antigens which react with IgM and IgG antibodies. Infect. Immun. 41, 331-338.

Odenthal-Schnittler, M., Tomavo, S., Becker, D., Dubremetz, J.-F., and Schwarz, R.T. [1992]. Evidence for N- and O-glycosylation in *Toxoplasma gondii*. Biochem Hoppe-Seyler in press.

Odenthal-Schnittler, M., Tomavo, S., Becker, D., Dubremetz, J.-F., and Schwarz, R.T. [1983]. Evidence for N-glycosylation of the *Toxoplasma gondii* surface protein p23. Manuscript in preparation.

Schwarz, R.T. and Datema, R. [1982]. The lipid pathway of protein glycosylation and its inhibitors: The biological significance of protein-bound carbohydrates. Adv. Carbohyd. Chem. Biochem 40, 287-379.

Schwarz, R.T. and Datema, R. [1984]. Inhibitors of trimming: new tools in glycoprotein research. Trends Biochem. Sci. 9, 32-34.

Schwarz, R.T., Mayor, S., Menon, A.K., and Cross, G.A.M. [1989]. Biosynthesis of the glycolipid membrane anchor of *Trypanosoma brucei* variant surface glycoproteins: involvement of Dol-P-Man. Biochem. Soc. Trans. 17, 746-748.

Sharma, C.B., Babczinski, P., Lehle, L., and Tanner, W. [1974]. The role of dolicholmonophosphate in glycoprotein biosynthesis in *Saccharomyces cerevisiae* Eur. J. Biochem. 46, 35-41.

Sharma, S.D., Mullenax, J., Araujo, F.G., Erlich, H.A., and Remington, J.S. [1983]. Western blot analysis of the antigens of *Toxoplasma gondii* recognized by human IgM and IgG antibodies. J. Immunol. 131: 977-983.

Sharon, N. [1975]. Complex Carbohydrates. Their Chemistry, Biosynthesis, and Functions. Chapter 4 (Carbohydrate-Peptide linkages) pp65-83; Addison-Wesley, London.

Sibley, L.D. and Sharma, S.D. [1987]. Ultrastructural localization of an intracellular *Toxoplasma gondii* protein that induces protection in mice. Infection and Immunity. 55, 2137-2141.

Striepen, B. [1991]. Der Antigenkomplex mit niedrigem Molekulargewicht von *Toxoplasma gondii* ist eine Familie von Glykosyl-Phosphatidylinositol-Lipiden. Diplomarbeit, University of Marburg.

Striepen, B, Tomavo, S., Dubremetz, J.-F., and Schwarz, R.T. [1992]. Identification and characterization of glycosyl-inositol phospholipids in *Toxoplasma gondii*. Biochem. Soc. Trans. 20, 296S.

Tomavo, S., Schwarz, R.T., and Dubremetz, J.F. [1989]. Evidence for glycosyl-phosphatidylinositol anchor of *Toxoplasma gondii* major surface antigens. Mol. Cell. Biol. 9, 4576-4580.

Tomavo, S., Dubremetz, J.-F., and Schwarz, R.T. [1992a]. A family of glycolipids from *Toxoplasma gondii*. Identification of candidate glycolipid precursor(s) for *Toxoplasma gondii* glycosylphosphatidylinositol membrane anchors. J. Biol. Chem. 267, 11721-11728.

Tomavo, S., Dubremetz, J.F., and Schwarz, R.T. [1992b]. Cell-free synthesis of glycolipid candidate precursor(s) for glycosyl-phosphatidylinositol anchors of *Toxoplasma gondii* surface proteins. Biochem. Soc. Trans. 20, 166S.

Tomavo, S., Dubremetz, J.-F., and Schwarz, R.T. [1992c]. Biosynthesis of glycolipid precursors for glycosyl-phosphatidylinositol membrane anchors in a *Toxoplasma gondii* cell-free system. J. Biol. Chem. in press.

Tomavo, S., Couvreur, G., Leriche, M.A., Sadak, A., Achbarou, A., Fortier, B., and Dubremetz, J.F., [1992d]. Immunolocalization of a 4.6 kD antigen of *T. gondii* that elicits an early IgM response upon primary infection. In preparation.

Tomavo, S., Dubremetz, J.-F., and Schwarz, R.T. [1992e]. Structural analysis of glycosyl-phosphatidylinositol membrane anchor of the *Toxoplasma gondii* tachyzoite surface glycoprotein gp23. Manuscript submitted.

Zinker, C.F. [1992]. Posttranslationale Modification des Oberflächenproteins P30 von *Toxoplasma gondii*. Diplomarbeit, University of Marburg.

Zinecker, C.F., Tomavo, S., Striepen, B., Dubremetz, J.-F., and Schwarz, R.T. [1992]. Posttranslational modification of the *Toxoplasma gondii* protein P30. Biochem. Hoppe-Seyler, in press.

IMMUNOLOGY
OF
TOXOPLASMA

ROLE OF P30 IN ATTACHMENT AND IMMUNITY TO *T. GONDII*

Lloyd H. Kasper, Imtiaz A. Khan, Kenneth H. Ely and Jose R. Mineo
Departments of Medicine (Neurology) and Microbiology
Dartmouth Medical School
Hanover, N.H.
USA 03755

P30 antigen of *T. gondii* : Immunology and Molecular Biology

Because of its adaptability to the laboratory, most work has focused on the tachyzoite stage of *T. gondii*. [reviewed in Kasper et al., 1992]. Of the several antigens recognized by the immune sera Ig fraction, the most prevalent has a Mr of 30Kd. Most work to date on the various toxoplasma antigens has concentrated on either the 30Kd (P30) or 22Kd (P22) proteins. Of the two, P30 is the major iodinated protein on a number of geographically diverse human and animal isolates of toxoplasma [Ware and Kasper, 1987]. Analysis of the gene encoding the P30 molecule show it to be highly conserved with only an 8 amino acid variation among tested strains. The P30 gene is single-copy and contains no introns [Burg et al, 1988]. This molecule comprises 3-5% of the total parasite protein and is a major component of the vesicular network within the parasitophorous vacuole [Sibley et al, 1986]. Intact intra- and extracellular parasites show a homogeneous distribution of P30; however, upon invasion of the host cell, most of the monoclonal antibody against P30 is shed from the tachyzoite [Dubremetz et al, 1985]. Mono- and polyclonal antibody against P30 is parasiticidal to extracellular *T. gondii* in the presence of serum complement [Kasper et al, 1987]. By competition binding assay, a single monoclonal directed against P30 can inhibit 25-30% of the specific binding of human immune serum to toxoplasma, sugesting that P30 is the most immunogenic constituent of the tachyzoite and that a single region of this molecule may contain most of the immunogenic activity. Our preliminary data (discussed below) further suggests that antibody of P30 inhibits parasite infection of host cells by over 85%.

One of the overall specific goals of our laboratory has been to rigorously characterize the host immune response to P30. Our data suggest that P30 is an important antigen in eliciting both a humoral and cellular host response.

NATO ASI Series, Vol. H 78
Toxoplasmosis
Edited by Judith E. Smith
© Springer-Verlag Berlin Heidelberg 1993

In humans, P30 induces high titer production of IFN-γ [Khan et al, 1988]. In the experimental murine model, P30 is able to induce near 100% protection against acute and chronic infection in mice when administered with the proper adjuvant. This protection is mediated by CD8+ T cells and can be adoptively transfered to the naive recipient [Khan et al, 1988]. Moreover, this protection is genetically restricted and highly antigen specific for the P30 molecule.

The ability of native P30 to protect mice against *T. gondii* infection.

We have now completed many of our proposed studies on the induction of protective immunity against toxoplasmosis in the experimental host. As discussed previously, the induction of protective immunity against acute and chronic toxoplasmosis can be achieved using P30. This protein when administered to outbred mice in the presence of the saponin Quil A is able to induce almost 100% protection aganst acute infection without evidence of chronic intracerebral cyst development. Similar observations were made in the more naturally resistant inbred A/J mouse as well as the naturally susceptible C57 strain. Adoptive transfer of immune splenocytes from immunized inbred. A/J mice conferred a significant level (p < 0.001) of protection against subsequent challenge. Phenotypic analysis in outbred as well as two different strains of inbred mice (A/J and C57) demonstrated that CD8+ T cells are selectively stimulated by this immunization protocol. T cell depletion studies using specific mAb directed at either CD3+ or CD8+ T cell phenotype followed by adoptive transfer failed to confer protective immunity whereas CD4+ depletion had no effect: this indicates that CD8+ T cells are responsible for host immunity. These cytotoxic CD8+ T cells produced high titers of IFN-gamma and above normal levels of IL-2. These antigen specific CD8+ T cells were directly parasiticidal against radiolabelled extracellular *T. gondii*. These studies further support the critical immune function of P30 antigen specific CD8+ T cells in host immunity against *T. gondii* infection [Khan, et al., 1991].

We are very interested in furthering our understanding of cytotoxic mechanisms. To examine the antigen specificity of this response, immune splenocytes from mice immunized with P30 were evaluated for their ability to lyse peritoneal macrophages infected with three different strains of *T. gondii*. Macrophages infected with either the RH or P wild type strain tachyzoites were lysed at varying effector to target (E:T) ratio by nylon wool non-adherent immune splenocytes, whereas macrophages infected with a P30 deficient mutant (B mutant) of the P strain were not. We have described the isolation and characterization of this and other P30 antigen deficient mutants earlier [Kasper, 1987]. The gene encoding P30 for the wild type and B mutant were amplified by the polymeraction. This revealed a nonsense mutation in the B mutant such that its primary translation product is predicted to be about two-thirds the size of the wild type P30 molecule. Monoclonal antibody depletion studies indicate that the cytotoxic effect of the immune splenocytes is mediated by the CD8+ T cell population. Peritoneal macrophages infected with the three different strains (RH, P wild type, B mutant) from mice genetically restricted were not lysed by the immune CD8+ effector cell population. A cloned line (C3) of P30 antigen specific CD8+ T cells exhibited significant cytotoxicity against syngeneic peritoneal macrophages infected with either the RH or P strain tachyzoites. There was no macrophage lysis observed by these CD8+ effector cells of either syngeneic macrophages, infected with the B mutant, or nonsyngeneic macrophages, infected with the three different tachyzoite strains. These studies indicate that although immune CD8+ T cells are able to kill extracellular *T. gondii*, there is significantly greater enhancement of this process when P30 antigen is presented in the context of MHC [Kasper, et al., 1992].

We have now furthered our observations on the cloned P30 antigen-specific T cells. Our current panel of P30 specific mouse T cells is comprised of both CD8+ and CD4+ phenotypes. Cytokine analysis of these clones indicates that most produce abundant quantities of IFN-gamma and IL-2 as determined by PCR, Northern blot and biologic assays. They are currently being evaluated for the production of a number of other critical cytokines including IL-4, IL-5, IL-6, IL-10, TNF-α,β, TGF-β and GM-CSF. By adoptive transfer studies, we have been able to confirm in two separate experiments that the C3 clone (CD8+, IFN-γ+) is able to confer 100% protection against lethal challenge (P<.001). Interestingly, preliminary review of surviving mice indicates that they are totally devoid of intracerebral cysts suggesting these cloned CD8+ T cells were protective against both acute and chronic infection. By comparison other P30 specific clones (CD4+) failed to confer significant protection against challenge despite their ability to produce high titer IFN-gamma which is believed to be the primary cytokine responsible for host immunity to *T. gondii*. We are now evaluating the role of accessory T cells in host protection using mAb depleted mice (anti- CD4+ and IFN-γ) that have been adoptively transfered with the C3 clone.

Interaction between host cell and parasite: Attachment.

Another concern in our laboratory is to further understand attachment which is the first interaction between parasite and host cell prior to penetration and invasion. Very little is known about those factors which mediate attachment between host cell and *T. gondii*. It has been suggested by Furtaldo et al, [1992] that laminin and laminin binding proteins of 14-16Kd and 60Kd are involved in attachment of tachyzoites to host cells. Cholesterol might be used for attachment, but this is yet to be documented [Pfefferkorn, 1990]. Recently, Smith and colleagues [Grimwood and Smith, 1992] have reported on the role of P30 in host cell invasion. Using a single mAb directed at P30, these authors were able to demonstrate a 37% decrease of host cell infection. Inhibition of infection was antigen specific, independent of parasite aggregation and correlated with antibody concentration. Our studies further these observations by characterizing the mechanism of parasite : host cell attachment.

Antibody to P30 blocks parasite invasion.

We have also begun a series of experiments to determine the functional role of the P30 molecule. Monoclonal and polyclonal, monospecific antibodies to P30 inhibit attachment to and invasion of human fibroblasts and murine enterocytes. This inhibitory effect on invasion is not due to agglutination, as an Fab' fragment from a polyclonal monospecific antibody to P30 also has this effect. Neither treatment with urea nor antisera raised to other surface proteins alters this effect. These latter findings indicate that this inhibitory activity is not likely to be due to steric hindrance or complexing of surface epitopes contiguous to P30. Infectivity of wild type (P30+) parasites (RH and PTg strain) is inhibited by 86% and 40% respectively with autologous, heat treated, strain specific mouse antisera, whereas infectivity of mutant parasites deficient in P30 (PTgB strain) is inhibited only 6% by its corresponding autologous mouse antisera. Mice infected perorally develop secretory intestinal IgA antibody to P30 that blocks parasite infection of mouse enterocytes. These data indicate that P30 is involved in attachment to and invasion of at least two different cell types from two different hosts.

References

Burg, J.L., Perelman, D., Kasper, L.H., Ware, P.L., and Boothroyd, J.C., [1988] Molecular analysis of the gene encoding the major surface antigen of *Toxoplasma gondii*, J. Immun. 141(10): p. 3584-3591.

Decoster, A., Darcy, F., Caron, A., and Capron, A., IgA antibodies against P30 as markers of congential and acute toxoplasmosis, Lancet 2(8620): 1104-1107, 1988.

Dubremetz, J.F., Rodriguez, C., and Ferreira, E. *Toxoplasma gondii:* Redistribution of Monoclonal Antibodies on Tachyzoites During Host Cell Invasion, Exp. Parasitol. 59(24): p. 24-32, 1985.

Furtado, G.C., Slowil, M., Kleinman, H.K., and Jointer, K.A. [1992]. "Laminin enhances binding of *Toxoplasma gondii* tachyzoites to J774 murine macrophage cells." Infect. Immun. 60: 2337-2342.

Grimwood, J., and Smith, J.E. [1992]. *Toxoplasma gondii*: The role of a 30 kDa surface protein in host cell invasion. Exp. Parasitol. 74, 106-111.

Kasper, L.H. and Boothroyd, J.C., Warren, K., and Agabian, N., Editor, *Toxoplasma gondii:* Immunology and Molecular Biology, in Immunobiology and Molecular Biology of Parasitic Diseases, 1992, Blackwell Scientific: Cambridge (In Press).

Kasper, L.H., Khan, I.A., Ely, K.H., Buelow, R. and Boothroyd, J.C., Antigen-specific (p30) mouse CD8+ T cells are cytotoxic against *Toxoplasma gondii* infected peritoneal macrophages, J. Immun. 148(5): p. 1493-1498, 1992.

Kasper, L.H., Isolation and characterization of a monoclonal anti-P30 antibody resistant mutant of *Toxoplasma gondii*, Parasite Immunology 9(4): p. 433-445, 1987.

Khan, I.A., Smith, K.A. and Kasper, L.H. Induction of antigen-specific parasiticidal cytotoxic T cell splenocytes by a major membrane protein (P30) of *Toxoplasma gondii*, J. Imm. 41(10): p. 3600-3605, 1988.

Khan, I.A., Eckel, M.E., Pfefferkorn, E.R., and Kasper, L.H.,
Production of gamma interferon by cultured human lymphocytes
stimulated with a purified membrane protein (P30) from *Toxoplasma
gondii*, J Infect Dis 157(5): p. 979-984, 1988.

Khan, I.A., Ely, K.H., and Kasper, L.H. A purified parasite antigen (p30)
mediates CD8+ T cell immunity against fatal *Toxoplasma gondii*
infection in mice J. Immun. 147(10): p. 3501-3506, 1991.

Pfefferkorn, E., Wyler, D.J., Editor., The cell biology of T. gondii, in
Modern Parasite Biology : Cellular Immunological and Molecular
Aspects, 1990, W.H. Freedman and Co: New York. p. 26-50.

Sibley, L.D., Krahenbuhl, J.L., Adams, G., Mike, W., and Weidner, E.,
Toxoplasma modifies macrophage phagosomes by secretion of a vesicular
network rich in surface proteins, The Journal of Cell Biology 103
(September): p. 867-874, 1986.

Ware, P.L., and Kasper, L.H. Strain-specific antigens of *Toxoplasma
gondii*, Infect Immun 55(3): p. 778-783, 1987.

SECRETORY IgA, ANTIBODY TO SAG1, H-2 CLASS I-RESTRICTED CD8[+] T-LYMPHOCYTES AND THE INT-1 LOCUS IN PROTECTION AGAINST *TOXOPLASMA GONDII*

Rima McLeod, M.D.[1,3], Douglas G. Mack, Ph.D.[1], Charles Brown, M.S.[1,2], and Emil Skamene, M.D., Ph.D.[4,1].
[1] Department of Medicine
Michael Reese Hospital and Medical Center
2929 S. Ellis
Chicago, IL 60616

Abstract

A murine model of peroral and congenital infection was developed to study protection against *Toxoplasma gondii* as infection is naturally acquired. Immunization with a temperature sensitive mutant (ts4) *T. gondii* was found to confer protection against peroral and congenital infection using this model. As it was possible to elicit a protective immune response against infection, immune mechanisms potentially important to protection in this model were characterized and correlates during human infections were sought.

Intestinal *T. gondii*-specific-secretory IgA was found in these perorally infected mice. Similarly, human *T. gondii*-specific-secretory IgA in whey was identified. This whey secretory IgA prevented infection of enterocytes *in vitro* and was used to define epitopes which elicited such protective antibody. Presence of secretory IgA antibody to proteins ≤ 46 kd which appeared to correlate with protection of enterocytes and antibody to affinity purified SAG1 (P30) could be demonstrated in whey. Mechanisms whereby protective whey blocked invasion of host cells by *T. gondii* included agglutination, but not complement dependent lysis. However, blocking of invasion also occurred with whey samples that did not agglutinate *T. gondii*, which suggested that there were *T. gondii* ligands for host cell receptors or adhesins that were blocked by secretory antibody. As presence of antibody to SAG1 in whey appeared to correlate with protection by whey against invasion of enterocytes,

---

[2] The University of Chicago
[3] The University of Illinois at Chicago
[4] McGill University

NATO ASI Series, Vol. H 78
Toxoplasmosis
Edited by Judith E. Smith
© Springer-Verlag Berlin Heidelberg 1993

and blocking by whey could occur without agglutination, collaboratively with Lloyd Kasper's laboratory, studies were performed using monoclonal and polyclonal, monospecific serum antibodies to SAG1, as well as SAG1 deficient *T. gondii* mutants. These studies demonstrated that SAG1 is important in, but not essential for, invasion of murine enterocytes and human fibroblasts. These data demonstrate that secretory IgA and serum IgG to SAG1 could contribute to a protective immune response by partially blocking initial host cell invasion by tachyzoites and that such antibodies can be elicited in a murine model and are present in acutely infected humans.

Genetic regulation of resistance to *T. gondii* parasitemia and subsequent cyst formation, found in this model of Me49 *Toxoplasma* infection, was associated with the H-2, Class I, L^d gene and was mediated by $CD8^+$ T cells. It was influenced by H-2, Class II interactions as well. The Ity/BCG/Lsh gene on mouse chromosome one also was found to make a minimal contribution to protection against cyst formation. The association of protection with an L^d gene product has provided a powerful tool for definition of biologically significant protective epitopes. In addition, it has broader implications as it also provides a unique experimental ligand-receptor system for understanding antigen processing and presentation. We are also using transgenic mice with human MHC genes with this model, as well as characterization of genetic restriction of human CTL *in vitro*, to define genetic restriction and epitopes of interest in potentially protective human immune responses to *T. gondii*. For example, the human HLA B27 gene (introduced as a transgene) did not protect otherwise susceptible $H-2^b$ mice.

In addition, using recombinant inbred mice, five genes were found to be important in survival following peroral infection. Those genes that could be identified using a linkage map included the H-2 complex, an unidentified gene associated with resistance to Ectromelia, and the INT-1 locus (a protooncogene on mouse chromosome 15).

Secretory antibody, serum antibody to SAG1 and class I $CD8^+$ T-lymphocytes, can contribute to protection against toxoplasmosis. The association of survival following peroral *T. gondii* infection and the INT1 locus, as well as blastogenesis of lymphocytes from uninfected individuals in response to *Toxoplasma* antigens, suggested that *T. gondii* might have superantigens. Studies are underway to determine whether *T. gondii* has superantigens. If *T.*

gondii does have superantigens, this could elicit harmful cytokine responses as well as provide a mechanism (e.g., clonal deletion) for the *T. gondii* antigen specific lymphocyte tolerance we found in infants with congenital toxoplasmosis.

Introduction

To better understand pathogenesis of toxoplasmosis and to characterize potentially protective immune responses, a murine model of peroral and congenital infection was developed. This has provided considerable insight into potentially protective epitopes and immune responses and data that raise the possibility that *T. gondii* has epitopes that are superantigen(s) which may elicit harmful cytokine responses. This data is described herein.

Murine Model Initially, a murine model of peroral and congenital *T. gondii* infection was developed [McLeod et al., 1984]. These experiments provided a model which resembled infections in immunocompetent and immunocompromised humans, acquired as this infection is naturally, i.e., perorally and congenitally (Tables 1 and 2, Figure 1). In this model, in perorally infected SWR/J mice, there were *T. gondii* specific IgG and IgM serum antibodies, *T. gondii* antigen responsive T lymphocytes and activated macrophages. There was marked suppression of lymphocyte response to mitogens. Immunization with the ts4 strain of *T. gondii* protected against peroral and congenital challenge using this model (Table 2).

Using this model, murine secretory IgA (3) was discovered (Figure 2, Table 3) and the epitopes such IgA recognized were identified [Mineo et al, submitted, Figure 4].

Similarly, secretory IgA in whey from humans which blocks *T. gondii* infection of enterocytes, was identified using an ELISA and western blotting [Table 4, Figures 3 to 5, Mack and McLeod, 1992, in press]. Epitopes associated with blocking activity of whey were protein and appeared to be associated with epitopes $\leq$ 46 kd (Table 4).

Agglutination, as well as other mechanisms appear to be operative in this inhibition by whey, but not complement dependent lysis. As SAG1 was one major epitope recognized by whey (Table 4) and such antibody was found to be present in whey by dot blot using affinity purified SAG1 (kindly provided by Lloyd Kasper; Mack, McLeod, in press (1992)], the effect of mAbs to SAG1, (as well as P22 and antisporozoite mAbs) were studied [Mineo et al., submitted]. Two anti SAG1 mAbs, a polyclonal, monospecific IgG to SAG1 and Fabs of this polyclonal IgG blocked infection [Mineo et al., submitted]. These experiments were performed collaboratively with J Smith (Leeds, England), L. Kasper and J. Mineo (Dartmouth, New Hampshire) using murine enterocytes, human fibroblasts and MBDK cells. The Fabs did not alter infection by a SAG1 minus mutant and Fabs of antibody to P22 had no effect [Mineo et al., submitted]. Mechanisms of attachment of SAG1 to host cell glycosylated receptors were studied and are discussed elsewhere [Mineo et al., submitted]. The data above indicate that SAG1 has the potential to elicit secretory IgA and serum IgG that may contribute to protection against initial infection of host cells by *T. gondii*. However, other epitopes must also be involved in invasion as SAG1 insufficient mutant tachyzoites (i.e. that have a stop codon at the gene which encodes the 200th amino acid of SAG1), bradyzoites, and sporozoites which do not have surface SAG1 can invade host cells.

Class I Restricted CD8 Lymphocytes As we developed this model we found that there was remarkable genetic variation in response to peroral *T. gondii* infection which regulated parasitemia, cyst number in brain, histopathology, immune responses and survival [Brown and McLeod, 1990; McLeod et al, 1984, 1989, 1989a] (Tables 5-9, Figures 6-7). The region of the MHC that encodes Class I glycoproteins, regulated cyst formation (Table 6). Class II genes also contributed to protection against cysts [Table 8, Brown and McLeod, 1990]. CD8+ T lymphocytes mediated this protection [Table 9, Brown and McLeod, 1990].

The genetic restriction was for the L^d encoded glycoprotein. Thus L^d must contain *T. gondii* specific peptide in its antigen presenting groove that selects a T cell receptor that is capable of protecting against parasitemia and cyst formation. This is an ideal model for determination of the critical protective peptide and the protein of which it is part. Beyond the major importance to understanding immunity to *T. gondii* in a biologically relevant system in which this peptide confers protection, this observation is fascinating as it presents the opportunity to gain truly novel insight into the fundamental biologic processess of intracellular protein/peptide transport. It provides the opportunity to determine how proteins/peptide(s) from a parasite that enters a host parasitophorous vacuole, traffic through the host cell cytoplasm and endoplasmic reticulum (interacting with self glycoproteins) and then are displayed on the host cell surface rendering the cell a target for CD8+ (probably cytolytic) lymphocytes. This observation can be extended to determine whether this *T. gondii* peptide, or other peptides from the protein of which it is part, associates with additional mouse and human class I and II glycoproteins. The genetic restriction these studies have uncovered also permits determination of whether transgenic human MHC molecules can convert a susceptible mouse to a resistant one. The human HLA B27 gene did not make susceptible ($H2^b$) mice resistant [Brown, David, Rendone and McLeod, in progress]. The method [Van Bleek and Nathenson, 1990; Falk et al., 1991] we are working with to isolate the peptide bound by the L^d glycoprotein can also be applied to human MHC molecules and CTL. Further, we have noted what appears to be increased frequency of severe congenital toxoplasmosis in Laotain and Phillipine infants [McAuley et al., submitted] and are interested in whether there may be a genetic susceptibility in humans related to MHC class I (or II) peptide recognition similar to that which we discovered in mice.

INT-1: Superantigen(s) and potentially harmful cytokines? There were five genes (Figure 7) associated with survival and there were statistically significant associations of survival with the H-2 complex, a gene regulating resistance to Ectromelia and an RFLP to the INT1 locus (a protooncogene which is an insertion site for mouse mammary tumor virus [MMTV], Table 10). MMTV's have long terminal repeats that encode superantigen(s) that result in V Beta deletions [Marrack, et al., 1991].

Because of this association and data which suggested that diminished survival might be associated with an overly exuberant immune response (Table 7) we looked for homologies between MMTV LTR ORF, other superantigens and *T. gondii* epitopes. There is a motif that appears in the MMTV LTR ORF, bacterial superantigens, and in SAG1 and GRA2 but not chymotrypsin, erythropoietin and not *T. gondii* NTPase [Ho, Meredith, McLeod, in progress]. We have found that *Toxoplasma* antigens can induce blastogenesis in naive human lymphocytes [Vogel, Mack, Rendone, and McLeod, in progress] and Kasper, Ely, and Kahn have found that SAG1 can induce blastogenesis in naive murine lymphocytes (personal communication). Histopathology in mice that die following peroral infection (susceptible) (Figure 1) is similar to that caused by excessive tumor necrosis factor production (which may be important in pathogenesis of a number of infections, e.g., cerebral malaria). We hypothesize that susceptible mice in our model do not have certain T cell receptor V Beta deletions and respond to the related *T. gondii* superantigen with harmful cytokine production. To test this hypothesis, we intend to determine whether *T. gondii* has superantigens which interact with particular T cell receptor V Beta chains, whether the consensus sequence (especially that of SAG1) binds to Class II molecules and whether ablation of cytokines such as TNF, TGF Beta, IL4, IL1, or IL10 can convert a mouse strain that is susceptible into one that is resistant.

Summary

Secretory IgA, serum antibody to SAG1, and Class I CD8+ T lymphocytes can contribute to protection against *Toxoplasma*. The association of survival with an RFLP for the INT1 locus and blastogenesis of lymphocytes from uninfected individuals in response to *T. gondii* antigens suggests that *T. gondii* may have superantigens.

Acknowledgements

This work was supported by grant AI19645 from NIH NIAID, TMP. We thank Ms. Diane Patton and Ms. Ellen Holfels for their assistance in preparation of this manuscript.

References

Brown, C.R., and McLeod, R. [1990]. Class I MHC genes and CD8+ T cells determine cyst number in *Toxoplasma gondii* infection. J. Immunol. 145: 3438-3441.

Falk, K., Rotzche, O., Stevanovic, S. Jung, G., and Rammensee, H.G. [1991]. Allele specific motifs revealed by sequencing of self peptides eluted from MHC Molecules. Nature 351: 290-6.

Mack, D., and McLeod, R. [1992]. Human *Toxoplasma gondii* - specific secretory IgA reduces *T. gondii* infection of enterocytes *in vitro*. J. Clin. Invest. October, 1992 (in press).

Marrack, P., Kushnir, E., and Kappler, J.W. [1991] A maternally inherited superantigen encoded by a mammary tumor virus. Nature (London) 349:524.

McLeod, R., Estes, R.G., Mack, D.G. and Cohen, H. [1984] Immune response of mice to ingested *Toxoplasma gondii*: a model of *Toxoplasma* infection acquired by ingestion. J. Inf. Dis. 149: 234-244.

McLeod, R., Frenkel, J.K., Estes, R.G., Mack, D.G., Eisenhauer, P., and Gibori, G., [1988] Subcutaneous and intestinal vaccination with tachyzoites of *Toxoplasma gondii* and acquisition of immunity to peroral and congenital *Toxoplasma* challenge. J. Immunol. 140: 1632-1637.

McLeod, R., and Mack, D. [1986]. Secretory IgA specific for *Toxoplasma gondii*. J. Immunol. 136: 2640-2643.

McLeod, R., Eisenhauer, P., Mack, D., Brown, C. Filice, G., and Spitalny, G., [1989]. Immune responses associated with early survival after peroral infection with *Toxoplasma gondii*. J. Immunol. 142: 3247-3255.

McLeod, R., Skamene, E., Brown, C.R., Eisenhauer, P.B., and Mack, D.G., [1989a] Genetic regulation of early survival and cyst number after peroral *Toxoplasma gondii* infection of AXB/BXA recombinant inbred and B10 congenic mic. J. Immunol 143: 3031-3034.

Van Bleek, G.M. and Nathensen, S.G., [1990] Isolation of an endogenously processed, immunodominant viral peptide from the class I H-2K^b molecule. Nature (London) 348: 213-16.

Table 1. Histopathologic findings in SWR/J mice infected perorally with the
Me49 strain of *T. gondii*. Reprinted with permission from McLeod, et al.,
[1984].

Time after infection	Findings in indicated tissue*					
	Lymph nodes	Spleen	Thymus	Liver	Lungs, heart	Brain
2 days	Normal, T+ to T++	Normal	Normal	Normal	ND	ND
1 week	EH+++, PC+++, T+	EH+++, PC+++, T+	Cortical atrophy, T+	N+, I++, T+	I+, T+	N+++, I++, T+++
2 weeks	EH+++, PC+++, T+	EH+++, PC+++, T+	Cortical atrophy, T+	N+, I+++, T+	ND	ND
1 month	EH++, PC+, T+	EH+++, PC+++	Normal	I++	ND	ND
2 and 4 months	EH+, PC+	PC+	Normal	I+	ND	ND
5 months	EH+, PC+	PC+	Normal	I+	I+	Cysts ++ to +++

*ND = not done; + = rare; ++ = few; +++ = many; T = toxoplasma
trophozoites observed in preparations stained by the *Toxoplasma*-specific
peroxidase-antiperoxidase technique; EH = epithelioid histiocytes; PC =
plasma cells; N = areas of necrosis; and I - Inflammation with collections of
mononuclear cells (especially around veins).

Table 2. Protection against peroral and congenital transmission by
immunization with a temperature sensitive mutant *T. gondii* tachyzoite (ts4) *T.
gondii*. Reprinted with permission from McLeod et al [1988].

A. Effect of immunizations on survival after s.c. challenge with tachyzoites of
the M7741 strain of *T. gondii*.

Immunization	No. of mice surviving challenge[a]				
	50[b]	100	200	1500	10.000
Sham intraintestinally	1/5 (20)	2/10 (20)	0/4 (0)	0/5 (0)	ND
Sham s.c.	3/5 (60)	2/10 (20)	1/5 (20)	0/5 (20)	ND
ts4 intraintestinally	4/5 (80)	7/10 (70)	1/5 (20)	1/5 (20)	ND
ts4 s.c.	ND	ND	ND	24/25 (96)	11/12 (92)

[a] Number of mice that survived challenge with M7741 tachyzoites. Numbers in parentheses, percentage of surviving mice.
[b] Number of tachyzoites used for challenge

B. Effect of immunization on numbers of brain cysts developing after peroral challenge.

Immunization	No. of mice[a] with		No. of cysts[b]		p value[c]
	≤3 cysts	>3 cysts	Mean ± SD	Range	
Control[d]	0	18	75 ± 48	14–163	NA[e]
ts4 s.c.	5	1	2 ± 3	0–9	0.002
Sham intraintestinal-ly[f]	0	5	68 ± 46	14–148	NA
ts4 intraintestinally[f]	2	6	18 ± 13	0–39	0.02

[a] Total number of mice is number with ≤3 cysts plus number with >3 cysts.
[b] At 30 days after peroral challenge with 200 cysts of the Me49 strain of *T. gondii*.
[c] Compared with control.
[d] Untreated mice age matched to those mice that received ts4 s.c.
[e] NA, not applicable.
[f] Performed at a different time from immunization and challenge of s.c. immunized mice.

C. Estimation of numbers of *Toxoplasma* in brains after peroral challenge, as determined by subinoculation of serial dilutions.

Immunization[b]	No. of Mice[a]		
	1/100[a]	1/1000	>1/10,000
Sham			12
ts4 s.c.	3	4	
ts4 intraintestinally	2	1	7

[a] Highest dilution of brain producing toxoplasma antibody titer ≥1/4 measured by Sabin-Feldman dye test in sera of recipient mice. Brain tissue was subinoculated after peroral challenge with 200 cysts of the Me49 strain of *T. gondii*.
[b] Subinoculated from nonpregnant mice at 30 days after challenge.

D. Fraction of infected mice in litters delivered by mice perorally challenged with the ME49 strain of *T. gondii* on the 11th day of gestation.

Immunization	Infected/Total[a]	Litters with ≥50% Infected Neonates[b,c]	Litters with 100% Infected Neonates[d]	Fraction of Litters Infected[e]
Sham intraintestinally	99/107 (93)	11/12 (92)	9/12 (75)	0.93 ± 0.16
Sham s.c.	47/53 (89)	6/7 (86)	6/7 (86)	0.91 ± 0.20
ts4 intraintestinally	74/115 (64)	13/16 (81)	8/16 (50)	0.69 ± 0.38
ts4 s.c.	86/91 (95)	7/7 (100)	5/7 (71)	0.94 ± 0.11

[a] Numerator, number of infected fetuses or neonates; denominator, total number of fetuses or neonates born to these mice. Numbers in parentheses, percentage.
[b] Numerator, number of litters with ≥50% infected neonates; denominator, total number of litters. Numbers in parentheses, percentage.
[c] Two dams in the sham intraintestinal treatment group and two dams in the ts4 intraintestinal treatment group were alive on the evening of the 18th day of gestation but dead on the morning of the 19th day of gestation.
[d] Numerator, number of litters with 100% infected neonates or fetuses; denominator, total number of litters. Numbers in parentheses, percentage.
[e] Mean ± SD.

Table 3. Murine Secretory IgA to *T. gondii*. Reprinted with permission from McLeod and Mack [1986].

A.

IgA to *T. Gondii* (measured by ELISA) in intestinal secretions of mice that received the Me49 strain of *T. Gondii* or cholera toxin[a]

Treatment of Mice and Secretions	Reciprocal of Dilution of Secretions[a]				
	10	40	160	640	2560
None	51	38	56	51	46
Cholera toxin perorally	43	47	54	49	44
Me49 cysts perorally	133	78	65	55	42
Me49 cysts perorally; secretions were absorbed with brain	'47	77	68	45	44
Me49 cysts perorally; secretions were absorbed with brain and tachyzoites of the RH strain of *T. Gondii*	64	43	48	53	40

[a] Values represent absorbance at 405 nm × 1000. Average of values obtained in duplicate wells.

B.

Time course of appearance of secretory IgA in intestinal secretions after peroral infection with the Me49 strain of *T. Gondii*

Mouse No.	Week after infection												
	0[a]	1	2	3	4[a]	5[b]	6	7	8	9	10	11	12
1					+[d]	0	+	0	0	0		0	
2						+	+	0	0		0	0	0
3					+	+	+	+	0[e]	0	0		0
4	0[c]								0[e]		0	0	0
5		0[c]			+	+	+	+	0			0	
6		0			+	+	+	+	0		0		

[a] Two hundred cysts administered perorally.

[b] Ten thousand cysts administered perorally to mice 1 and 2 and 2000 cysts administered perorally to mice 3 to 6. Mice 1 and 2 received the same inocula at the same time in the first experiment, as did mice 3 and 4 in the second experiment, and mice 5 and 6 in the third experiment. Secretions from two uninfected mice were collected and analyzed at the same times as those from the two infected mice in each experiment.

[c] 0 = No IgA was found in secretions by using the ELISA; i.e., the absorbance at 405 nm of a fourfold or smaller dilution of secretions was less than twice the absorbance of secretions from the two uninfected mice studied at the same time. Two mice at 8 wk (indicated by e) had IgA in undiluted or fourfold dilution of intestinal secretions, and all the others were negative in undiluted or fourfold dilutions of secretions.

[d] + = IgA was found in secretions by using the ELISA; i.e., the absorbance at 405 nm of an eightfold or greater dilution of secretions was twice the absorbance of secretions from the two uninfected mice studied at the same time.

[e] Explanation contained in footnote c.

Table 4. Clinical status of human whey donors (A) and correlation of *T. gondii* secretory IgA epitopes with inhibition by whey of subsequent replication of *T. gondii* in enterocytes (B). Reprinted with permission from Mack and McLeod, [1992].

A. Serologic test results for women from whom whey was obtained.

Status of Infection	Subject Number	Infant DOB	Estimate of Trimester of Acquisition	Date Sera Obtained	Date Milk Obtained	Reciprocal of Serum Dye Test*	Serum IgM ELISA*	Serum IgA ELISA*	Serum AC/HS*
Acute	1	11/90	second	9/90	11/90	8000	7.7	9.4	>1600/1600
Acute	2	10/90	third	11/90	11/90	1024	3.9	5.6	>1600/3200
Acute	3	3/89	third	7/89	5/89	4096	4.8	not done	>1600/3200
Acute	17	1/91	third	4/91	4/91	8000	10.8	not done	>1600/3200
Subacute	4†	8/90	periconceptual	11/90	11/90	256	3.0	5.6	400/800
Chronic	5	7/89	not applicable	9/89	9/89	512	0.2	not done	not done
Chronic	6	9/90	not applicable	11/90	11/90	positive§	negative§	not done	not done
Chronic	7	1/91	not applicable	2/91	1/91	512	0.5	not done	50/3200
Chronic	8	1/91	not applicable	1/89	2/91	1024	1.6	not done	not done
Chronic	9	12/90	not applicable	6/87	1/91	16000	1.6	not done	not done
Chronic	10	11/90	not applicable	12/90	12/90	64	0.1	not done	not done
Chronic	11	10/90	not applicable	10/90	11/90	32	0.4	not done	not done
Uninfected	12	7/90	not applicable	10/90	11/90	negative	not done	not done	not done
Uninfected	13	9/90	not applicable	11/90	1/91	negative	not done	not done	not done
Uninfected	14	3/90	not applicable	1/90	10/90	negative	not done	not done	not done
Uninfected	15	12/89	not applicable	10/90	10/90	negative	not done	not done	not done
Uninfected	16	3/89	not applicable	9/89	9/89	negative	not done	not done	not done

* At the time milk sample was obtained; AC/HS refers to the "Differential agglutination" test of Desmonts, Thulliez and Remington. This test uses acetone (AC) and formalin (HS) fixed tachyzoites. It is useful in determining whether infection was acquired in the 6 months prior to the time when the serum sample was obtained. The results for the acutely and subacutely infected women demonstrate that their infections were recently acquired.
† Treated with spiramycin during gestation.
§ IgG by EIA, IgM by IFA

B. Correlation of presence of *T. gondii* specific secretory IgA in ELISA, Epitopes recognized in western blots and inhibitory effect of whey on subsequent replication of *T. gondii* in enterocytes.

Molecular Weight of Epitope	Acute				Subacute/Chronic								Uninfected				
	1*	2	3†	17	4§	5	6	7	8	9	10	11	12	13	14	15	16
>100	+	+	+				±	+	+	+							
69-92	+ +	+ +	+		+		+	+									
46-69	+	+	+	+		+											
46	+	+	+	+		+	+	+									
30	+ +	+ +	+ +	±													
21-30			+ +														
22	±	±	+														
≤14	+	+	+														
T. gondii specific ELISA results (OD)	917	642	266	not done	25	64	78	69	134	115	61	1	111	42	¶	65	58
Percent Inhibition‖	>75	50	50	not done	0	50	40	40	15	15	0	0	0	0	0	0	0

++ = strongly positive, + = present, ± = equivocal
* Subject number
† This whey sample also contained secretory IgA which recognized epitopes between 14 and 22 kd.
§ Treated with Spiramycin during gestation.
¶ Whey from this seronegative mother had nonspecific reactivity in some assays.
‖ Percent Inhibition = percent inhibition of T. gondii infection of enterocytes due to whey. Inhibition appeared to correlate with presence of T. gondii secretory IgA to epitopes ≤46kd demonstrated in Western blots.

Table 5. Histopathologic findings in A/J and C57BL/6J mice infected perorally with the Me49 strain of *T. gondii*. Adapted with permission from McLeod et al [1989].

Strain of Mouse	Time after infection (Days)	Findings in Indicated Tissue				
		Mesenteric nodes	Liver	Lung	Heart	Brain
A/J	3	NS[a]	NS	NS	NS	I[+]
A/J	7	EM[+++], K[++], NB[+], LD[+++], T[+]	I[++], EM[+++], K[+], N[++]	NS	NS	I[+], N[+]
C57BL/6J	3	EM[++]	I[++], N[++]	NS	NS	I[+]
C57BL/6J	7	EM[+++], K[+++], NB[++], N[+], LD[+++], T[++]	I[+++], EM[+++], K[++], N[+++], vacuolated hepatocytes	1 mouse, NS; 2nd mouse, small foci of acute pneumonia	NS	I[++]

[a] NS, no significant findings compared to controls; +, rare; ++, few; +++, many; T, *Toxoplasma* tachyzoites observed in preparations stained by the Toxoplasma-specific peroxidase-antiperoxidase technique; EM, epithelioid macrophages; K, karyorrhexis, NB, necrobiosis, N, areas of necrosis; LD, areas of lymphocyte depletion; and I, inflammation.

Table 6. Effect of peroral *T. gondii* infection on splenic lymphocyte subsets. Adapted with permission from McLeod et al. [1989].

Strain of Mouse	Day of Infection	% Lyt-2	% L3T4
A/J	Uninfected	8 ± 2.4[a]	22 ± 7.4[b]
	3	9.8 ± 1.9	20.2 ± 4.7
	7	7.8 ± 2.8	9.7 ± 3.4
C57BL/6	Uninfected	12.2 ± 3.3	24.3 ± 4.2
	3	11.3 ± 2.8	20.1 ± 7.2
	7	8.4 ± 1.2	6 ± 4[b]

[a] Mean ± SD; n = six to eight mice per group.

[b] The differences that achieved statistical significance were: % Lyt-2 lymphocytes from uninfected C57BL/6 and C57BL/6 mice at 7 days after infection (p = 0.02); % L3T4 lymphocytes of both strains of mice on the 7th day after infection compared with those from uninfected mice (C57BL/6, p < 0.0001; A/J, p < 0.004.) % L3T4 cells from A/J and C57BL/6 mice 7 days after infection were not significantly different (p = 0.2).

Table 7. Comparison of histopathology and immune responses after peroral _Toxoplasma_ challenge of C57BL/6 and A/J mice. Adapted with permission from McLeod, et al [1989].

Parameter Studied	Result for Strain of Mouse	
	C57BL/6	A/J
T. gondii in blood, liver, and brain	Greater numbers	Smaller numbers
Challenge followed by sulfadiazine therapy	Sulfadiazine protects	Protected with and without sulfadiazine therapy
Administration of formalin-treated RH	Not lethal	Not lethal
Resistance to i.p. relative to peroral infection	Greater than peroral	Resistant to both i.p. and peroral infection
Histopathology	More necrosis and inflammation	Minimal necrosis and inflammation
% Splenic Lyt-2⁺ lymphocytes	Greater decrease	Decrease
% Splenic L3T4⁺ lymphocytes	Same decrease	Same decrease
Lymphocyte blastogenic response to Con A after infection	Greater decrease	Decrease
Lymphocyte IFN-γ production unstimulated after peroral infection	Increase	No increase
Lymphocyte IFN-γ production after stimulation in vitro with _Toxoplasma_ Ag	Increase, greater than for A/J mice	Increase
Serum IFN-γ levels after peroral infection	Increase	No increase from infection; levels higher than in C57BL/6 mice
IL-2 production in vitro	Same increase	Same increase
Serum IgG antibody measured with Sabin-Feldman dye test	Same increase	Same increase
Serum _Toxoplasma_-specific IgM	Smaller increase	Increase
Peritoneal macrophage microbicidal capacity	No activation when mice are uninfected or 3 days after infection; enhanced 7 days after infection	Same as for C57BL/6 mice
Kupffer cell microbicidal capacity after peroral infection	Increase	No increase

Table 8. Effect of H-2 haplotype and mutations in H-2 on cyst formation following peroral infection with _T. gondii_ bradyzoites[a]. Adapted with permission from Brown and McLeod [1990].

	H-2 Haplotype									Cyst Number	
Strain	K	A	E	D	L	Qa-2	TLA	Qa-1	_n_	Mean±SD	Range
C57BL/6J	b	b	b	b	b	a	b	b	15	49±40	14-178
A/J	k	k	k	d	d	a	a	a	24	1±1	0-3
BALB/c	d	d	d	d	d	b	c	b	8	2±1	0-4
C57BL/10SnJ	b	b	b	b	b	a	b	b	16	60±32	20-141
B10.A/SgSnJ	k	k	k	d	d	a	a	a	31	2±2	0-8
B10.A(4R)	k	k	b	b	b	a	b	b	11	83±31	38-131
B10.A(2R)	k	k	k	b	b	a	b	b	12	48±43	15-175
B10.BAR6	k	k	k	b	b	•	•	•	11	60±25	17-96
B10.BAR12	b	b	b	d	d	•	•	•	12	2±1	0-4
B10.MBR	b	k	k	q	q	a	a	a	16	75±36	34-170
B10.D2-H-2dm1	d	d	d	(d)	(d)	•	•	•	12	315±277	84-796
BALB/c-H-2dm2	d	d	d	d	–	b	c	b	7	341±115	160-461
B6.C-H-2bm12	b	(b)	b	b	b	•	•	•	17	151±92	47-458

[a]_n_, number of mice in two or three experiments. •, allele at this locus has not been defined. --, loss of the L^d gene. All mice had antibodies to _T. gondii_ 30 days after peroral infection. Mice that were H-2L^b had significantly more cysts ($p < 0.001$). Mice with mutations in A and L had significantly more cysts ($p < 0.001$).

Table 9. Effect of depletion of CD8+ lymphocytes *in vivo* on cyst formation after peroral infection of B10.BAR6 and 12 mice. Adapted with permission from Brown and McLeod [1990].

| Strain | Antibody | n* | Cyst number | |
			Mean ± SD	Range
B10.BAR6	G16/1	6	58±40	16-126
	YTS169.4	12	82±65	14-235
B10.BAR12	G16/1	8	3±4	0-12
	YTS169.4	14	95±52	31-144

* Number of mice. YTS169.4 mice were depleted
of >95% of their CD8+ T-cells on days 3, 9 and 18
after administration.

Table 10. Association of INT-1 locus RFLP on mouse chromosome 15 and survival following peroral infection with the Me49 strain of *T. gondii* in AXB/BXA recombinant inbred mice.

| INT1 LOCUS | MEAN DAYS OF SURVIVAL AFTER PERORAL INFECTION | |
	<20	>20
a/a	0[a]	11[a]
b/b	4[a]	5[a]

a Number of mouse strains. There were a minimum of 5 mice of each of the 20 recombinant inbred strains typed in each experiment and each experiment was performed at least twice. Differences between Int 1 a/a and b/b mouse strains were significant, p = 0.026 when tested by Fisher Exact test and Z = 1.96 (p < 0.05) when tested using Briles analysis and a linkage map.

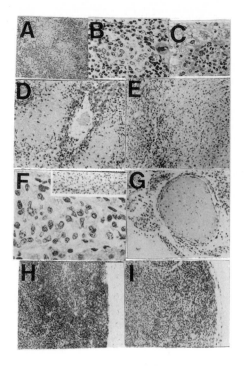

<u>Figure 1</u>. Histopathology during peroral infection of resistant and susceptible mice. Lesions in hemtoxylin and eosin stained lymphoid tissues and livers of SWR/J mice given the Me49 strain of *T. gondii* perorally (A-C). A. Epithelioid cells in lymph node from a mouse infected 13 days earlier. Large foci of macrophages without the formation of definite nodules are apparent. B. Spleen tissue from a mouse infected 27 days earlier. A cluster of epithelioid cells is visible. C. Liver tissue from a mouse infected 72 days earlier. An inflammatory focus is evident in a lobule. Small and large lymphocytes and degenerating hepatic cells are also seen, as is one mitosis. Tissues from Beige and C57BL/6J mice infected with the Me49 strain of Toxoplasma (D-G). D. Beige mouse. A large focus of necrosis is seen on either side of a vein. E. C57 Bl/6J mouse. Lymph node. A large focus of necrosis (arrow) is apparent in the cortex. F. Liver from a Beige mouse. The lumen of a vein is filled with monohistiocytic cells. Vessel wall is shown in the inset at lower magnification. G. Lymph node tissue from a C57BL/6J mouse. A large vein and artery are filled with thrombi. Interestingly, in both groups of mice there was marked loss of thymic cortical tissue. H. Uninfected control SWR/J thymus. I. SWR/J mouse thymus 13 days after peroral infection. Note loss of thymic cortical tissue. Reprinted with permission from McLeod, et al [1984].

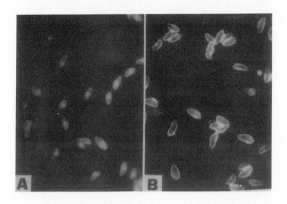

Figure 2. Immunofluorescent assay that demonstrates IgA specific for *T. gondii.*

A. Tachyzoites of the RH strain of *T. gondii* incubated with intestinal secretions from mice that received uninfected mouse brain perorally.

B. Tachyzoites of the RH strain of *T. gondii* incubated with intestinal secretions from mice infected with brain that contained bradyzoites of the Me49 strain of *T. gondii* perorally. Note immunofluorescence around perimeter of the tachyzoites. (Reprinted with permission from McLeod and Mack [1986].

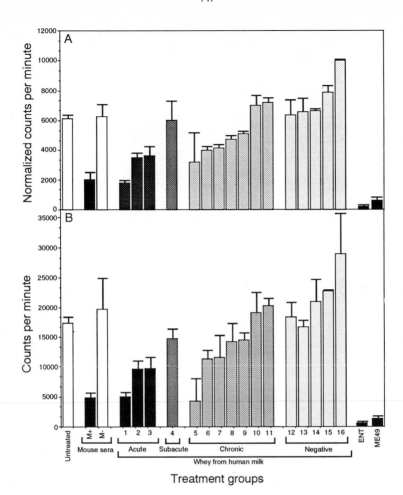

Figure 3. Effect of treatment (incubation) of tachyzoites with whey from sixteen women on Me49 strain T. gondii infection of enterocytes in vitro. A. These are normalized data pooled from at least 2 representative experiments. B. Representative experiments, CPM. Numbers are the same as used in other Tables and Figures to indicate whey from individual subjects. Differences between whey from uninfected and infected individuals were signficant ($p < 0.05$). Untreated refers to enterocytes cultured with media alone. MS = mouse sera. M+ = treatment with sera from infected mice; M- = sera from uninfected mice; Acute = treatment with whey from acutely infected woman; Subacute = treatment with whey from subacutely infected woman; Chronic = treated with whey from chronically infected woman; Negative = treatment with whey from uninfected woman. ENT refers to CPM from enterocytes in culture alone; Me49 refers to CPM from the Me49 strain of *T. gondii* in culture alone. Reprinted with permission from Mack and McLeod (1992).

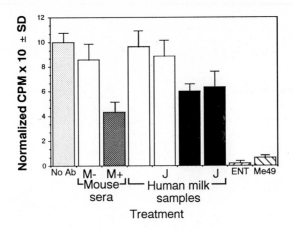

Figure 4. Effect of whey, secretory IgA isolated from whey using a jacalin affinity column, and mouse sera on the subsequent replication of Me49 strain T. gondii tachyzoites in enterocytes challenged in vitro. ▨ Represents effect of media alone. □ represents effect of sera from the seronegative mice or whey or secretory IgA isolated from this whey (whey, jacalin [J]) from the seronegative mother. ▨ represents the effect of serum from the chronically infected mouse and ■ the effect of whey, or secretory IgA isolated from this milk (whey, jacalin) from the acutely infected woman. Dilutions of mouse sera were 1:10 and whey 1:2. The sera from the infected mouse and milk and IgA from the infected individual significantly reduced CPM ($p < 0.05$). Reprinted with permission from Mack and McLeod, (1992).

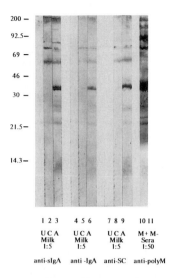

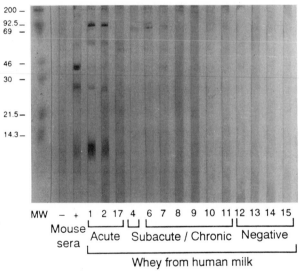

Figure 5. Epitopes recognized by human secretory IgA. TOP. Western blots which indicate molecular weights of antigens *T. gondii* recognized by human whey. U = whey from initially studied uninfected woman (number 16); C = whey from initially studied chronically infected woman (number 5); A = whey from initially studied actuely infected woman (number 3). Antigens are those recognized when probed with antibody to secretory IgA (anti SIgA), IgA (Anti IgA) and secretory piece (anti SC). Sera from infected (M+) and uninfected mice (M-) controls were probed with antibody to mouse immunoglobulin (anti-poly).
BOTTOM. Western blots with whey from the other 14 women. There was a very faint band at 30 kd for number 17 which is not seen in this photograph. Reprinted with permission from Mack and McLeod (1992).

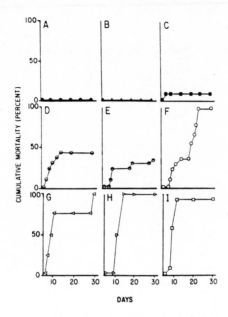

Figure 6. Survival of inbred mouse strains following peroral *T. gondii* infection. The numbers and strains of mice tested were A, 10 A/J: B, 8 C3H/HeJ: C, 11 DBA2/J: D, 11 DBA1/J; E, 12 BALB/c BYJ: F, 11 C57L/J: G, 4 SJL/J: H, 4 SB/LE: and I, 18 C57BL/6J. Reprinted with permission from McLeod et al [1989].

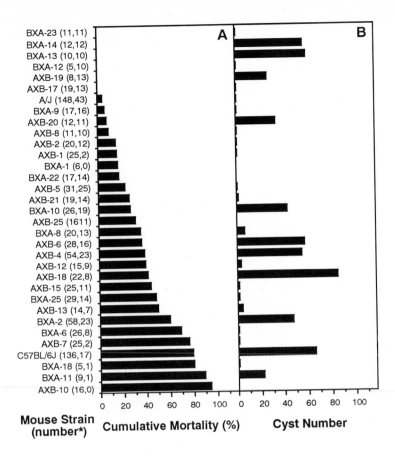

Figure 7. Cumulative mortality (A) and cyst number (B) 30 days after peroral infection of AXB and BXA recombinant inbred strains of mice. *The first number within parentheses represents the number of mice studied for mortality. The second number within parentheses represents the number of mice studied for brain cyst number. Adapted with permission from McLeod et al [1989a].

FACTORS RESPONSIBLE FOR DEVELOPMENT OF TOXOPLASMIC ENCHEPHALITIS IN IMMUNOCOMPROMISED HOSTS

Yasuhiro Suzuki
Department of Parasitology
Jikei University School of Medicine
3-25-8 Nishi-Shinbashi, Minato-Ku
Tokyo 105
Japan

Toxoplasmic encephalitis has emerged as a major cause of morbidity and mortality in patients with AIDS [Levy *et al.* 1985; Luft and Remington 1988]. Before the advent of AIDS, this encephalitis was rarely diagnosed in adults. In patients infected with HIV, the encephalitis occurs almost solely in individuals with preexisiting antibodies to *Toxoplasma* [Luft *et al.* 1984; Wong *et al.* 1984]. Thus, encephalitis appears to be caused by recrudescence of a previously latent *Toxoplasma* infection. It is unknown whether the original site of recrudescence is the brain itself or extraneural with haematogenous spread to the brain. In most cases the CD4 counts are well below 100 / cumm.

Toxoplasmic encephalitis develops in 5% to 10% of AIDS patients in the United States and 25% to 50% of AIDS patients in Europe. The cause of this striking difference appears to be the greater prevalence of latent Toxoplasma infection in much of western Europe. AIDS patients in (or from) tropical countries should be considered at especially high risk. The reason again is presumably the greater prevalence of the latent infection. WHO estimated in 1991 that the number of AIDS patients will reach 10 million in the world by the year 2000. This estimate gives us a warning that hundreds of thousands of cases of toxoplasmic encephalitis will occur in AIDS patients in the near future if preventive measures are not found.

The fact that toxoplasmic encephalitis is often observed in immunocompromised patients in clear contrast to immunologically normal individuals indicates that the immune system plays a critically important role in the prevention of this disease. To analyze how the immunologically normal host maintains the chronic (latent) nature of the infection without suffering the encephalitis is critical to our understanding of the pathogenesis of this disease. Toward this

NATO ASI Series, Vol. H 78
Toxoplasmosis
Edited by Judith E. Smith
© Springer-Verlag Berlin Heidelberg 1993

end, we have employed murine models of toxoplasmic encephalitis in an attempt to identify the mechanism(s) operative in both prevention and recrudescence of the latent infection in the central nervous system.

Importance of endogenous IFN-γ for prevention of toxoplasmic encephalitis.

Neutralization of endogenous IFN-γ in chronically infected mice, by using a monoclonal antibody (mAb) to this lymphokine, induced severe inflammatory changes in their brains [Suzuki et al. 1989]. Control mice that received saline or normal IgG had slight inflammation in their brains. In contrast to control mice, the mAb-treated mice had many areas of acute focal inflammation and infiltration of large numbers of inflammatory cells in the meninges and parenchyma of their brains. In the areas of acute focal inflammation, the presence of tachyzoites and toxoplasma antigens were demonstrated by immunoperoxidase staining with the use of anti-toxoplasma antibody, suggesting that the focal inflammation was induced by proliferation of tachyzoites. Acute inflammation was also observed around cysts of *T. gondii*. Immunohistologic staining revealed tachyzoites and toxoplasma antigens surrounding the periphery of these cysts, suggesting cyst disruption had occurred. These results suggest that IFN-γ plays a critical role in preventing cyst rupture and toxoplasmic encephalitis. Impairment of IFN-γ production in AIDS patients [Murray et al. 1984] is probably a major factor in predisposing to the high incidence of the encephalitis in these patients. The mechanisims (s) by which IFN-γ prevents cyst rupture require further study.

Effect of genetic background of host on development of toxoplasmic encephalitis.

It is known that resistance against acute infection [Araujo et al. 1976; Williams et al. 1978] and formation of cysts in the brain of mice [Jones and Erb 1985; Brown and McLeod 1990] are genetically controlled. The fact that at least 30% of AIDS patients who have antibodies to *T.gondii* will develop toxoplasmic encephalitis [Luft and Remington 1988] raises the possibility that host genetic differences may contribute to the development and severity of the clinical manifestation of the encephalitis. In a mouse model, mice with the H-2^b and H-2^k haplotypes developed remarkable inflammatory changes in their brains during chronic infection with the ME49 strain of *T.gondii* whereas mice with the H-2^a and H-2^d haplotypes did not [Suzuki *et al.* 1991]. An analysis using B10 congenic mice revealed that a gene(s) within the H-2D region controls the development of the encephalitis. Whether similar genetic regulation may be operative in determining development of toxoplasmic encephalitis in patients with AIDS is not known.

Effect of strains of *Toxoplasma gondii* on development of toxoplasmic encephalitis

The strain of *T.gondii* also appears to be a critical factor in the development of inflammatory responses in the brain during chronic infection. For example, both the DAG and ME49 strains are avirulent in CBA/Ca mice (H-2^k haplotype) during the acute stage of infection. However, during the chronic stage of infection, only the ME49 strain induced remarkable inflammatory changes in the brain [Suzuki *et al.* 1988].

Chronic infection in C57BL/10 mice (H-2^b haplotype) with either the C56 or Beverley strain induced no inflammatory responses in their brain. There was no difference in the number of cysts per brain between mice infected with the C56 and Beverley strains. However, after treatment of those mice with anti-IFN-γ mAb, remarkable inflammatory changes were induced only in the brains of mice infected with the Beverley strain (unpublished data).

References

Araujo, F.G., Williams, D.M., Grument, F.C., Remington, J.S. (1976) Strain-dependent differences in murine susceptibility to Toxoplasma. Infect Immun 13:1528-1530.

Brown, C.R., McLeod, R. (1990) Class I MHC genes and CD8$^+$ T cells determine cyst number in *Toxoplasma gondii* infection. J Immunol 145:3438-3441.

Jones, T.C., Erb, P. (1985) H-2 complex-linked resistance in murine toxoplasmosis. J Infect Dis 151:739-740.

Levy, R.M., Bredensen, B.E., Rosenblum, M.L. (1985) Neurological manifestations of the acquired immunodeficiency syndrome (AIDS): experience at UCSF and review of the literature. J Neurosurg 162: 475-495.

Luft, B.J., Brooks, R.G., Conley, F.K., McCabe, R.E., Remington, J.S. (1984) Toxoplasmic encephalitis in patients with AIDS. JAMA, 252:913-917.

Luft, B.J., Remington, J.S. (1988) AIDS commentary; Toxoplasmic encephalitis. J Infect Dis 157:1-6.

Murray, H.W., Rubin, B.Y., Masur, H., Roberto, R.B. (1984) Impaired production of lymphokines and immune (gamma) interferon in the acquired immunodeficiency syndrome. N Engl J Med 310:883-889.

Suzuki, Y., Conley, F.K., Remington, J.S. (1988) Differences in virulence and development of encephalitis during chronic infection vary with the strain of *Toxoplasma gondii*. J Infect Dis 159:790-794.

Suzuki, Y., Conley, F.K., Remington, J.S. (1989) Importance of endogenous IFN-γ for prevention of toxoplasmic encephalitis in mice. J Immunol 143:2045-2050.

Suzuki, Y., Joh, K., Orellana, M.A., Conley, F.K., Remington, J.S. (1991) A gene(s) within the H-2D region determines the development of toxoplasmic encephalitis in mice. Immunology 74:732-739.

Williams. D.M., Grumet, F.C., Remington, J.S. (1978) Genetic control of murine resistance to *Toxoplasma gondii*. Infect Immun 19: 416-420.

Wong, B., Gold, J.N.W., Brown, A.E., Lange, M., Fried, R., Grieco, M., Midvan, D., Giron, J., Tapper, M.L., Lerner, C.W., Armstrong, D. (1984) Central nervous system toxoplasmosis in homosexual men and parenteral drug abusers. Ann Intern Med 100:36-42.

SYNERGISTIC AND COMPENSATORY ROLES OF CD4+, CD8+ T-LYMPHOCYTES AND NATURAL KILLER CELLS IN RESISTANCE TO *TOXOPLASMA GONDII*

A. Sher, R.T.Gazzinelli, & E.Y.Denkers
Immunology and Cell Biology Section
Laboratory of Parasitic Diseases
National Institute of Allergy and Infectious Disease
Bethesda, Maryland 20892
U.S.A.

Cell-mediated immunity has long been recognized to play a crucial role in resistance to *Toxoplasma gondii*. Nevertheless, it is only within recent years that the events involved in cellular control of acute and chronic infection have begun to be defined. An important breakthrough occurred when Suzuki and Remington [Suzuki et al 1988] discovered the central role played by IFN-γ in resistance to new infection as well as in the control of re-activation. While the key effector function of this cytokine has now been confirmed, its mechanism of action remains poorly understood.

When spleen cells from infected mice or mice vaccinated with the ts-4 mutant are stimulated *in vitro* with toxoplasma antigens or mitogen, most of the IFN-γ produced is derived from CD4+ T lymphocytes [Gazzinelli et al 1991, 1992]. Nevertheless, depletion studies performed in both animal models reveal that removal of CD4+ cells fails to ablate resistance. Simultaneous depletion of CD8+ cells, which produce much smaller quantities of the cytokine *in vitro*, is necessary for full ablation. Moreover, in the vaccine model, a highly significant loss of resistance occurs in mice depleted of CD8+ cells alone. However, when mice are treated with anti-CD4+ antibodies during as opposed to after vaccination, they fail to display immunity to challenge [Gazzinelli, et al 1991].

These findings are consistent with the hypothesis (Figure 1) that CD4+ cells are not the major effector cells of resistance to *T. gondii in vivo*, but instead their major role is to provide helper function (presumably in the form of IL-2) to CD8+ effector cells or to act as a secondary source of IFN-γ. The reason why CD4+ lymphocytes, which produce high levels of IFN-γ *in vitro*, are not sufficient to mediate protection *in vivo* is not clear, but may relate to the

NATO ASI Series, Vol. H 78
Toxoplasmosis
Edited by Judith E. Smith
© Springer-Verlag Berlin Heidelberg 1993

preferential triggering of CD8+ cells by class I MHC bearing toxoplasma infected cells.

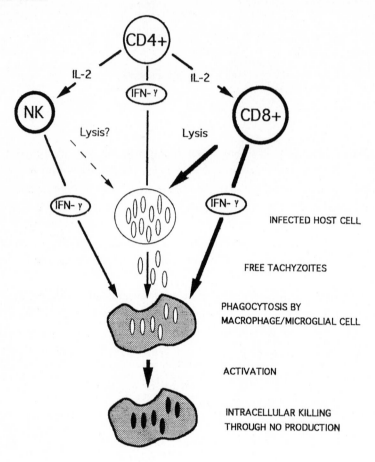

Figure 1. Proposed scheme for the interplay of CD4+, CD8+ lymphocytes and NK cells in resistance to *Toxoplasma gondii*

A second hypothesis is that the potent *in vivo* activity of CD8+ cells relates to their cytolytic function. It is now evident from several recent studies [Hakim *et al* 1991, Subauste *et al* 1991] that CD8+ cells from resistant mice can lyse *T. gondii* infected targets *in vitro*. If this effector function is also necessary for immunity *in vivo* it would explain the preferential requirement for CD8+ cells. As outlined in Figure 1, IFN-γ would then fit into the scheme as a cytokine needed for activation of macrophages to kill phagocytosed tachyzoites released as a consequence of host cell lysis. CD8+, CD4+, as well as NK cells (see below) could serve as a lymphokine source.

The importance of CD8+ lymphocytes as effector cells of resistance has stimulated considerable interest in identifying both their target epitopes in the parasite as well as the mechanisms by which these epitopes are processed and presented. A particularly useful experimental system for this work is the bone-marrow derived mcacrophage (BMDM) host target assay originally described by Hakim *et al* [1991]. In this procedure, BMDM, which express high levels of class I MHC products, can be made into targets for CD8+ CTL from vaccinated mice by either *T. gondii* infection or by incubation with parasite macromolecules (presumably proteins). The latter sensitization route allows for direct identification (by fractionation of the extract) of CTL target antigens. As revealed by recent studies (E.Y. Denkers *et al*, submitted), BMDM appear to process exogenously presented parasite antigen by an endogenous pathway and the resulting target epitopes cross-react with those presented by *T. gondii* infected BMDM. Thus, the CTL target molecules identified by this assay should be closely related to those seen on naturally infected cells. Recently developed techniques for isolating processed foreign peptides from MHC molecules offer a second strategy for CTL target epitope identification.

In order to confirm the role of CD8+ cells in protective immunity, we have recently tested the ability of β-2 microglobulin "knock-out" mice to develop vaccine (ts-4) induced resistance. These animals have inactivated β-2 microglobulin genes and consequently fail to make functional class I molecules. Because of this defect they show a near complete absence of CD8+ cells [Koller *et al* 1990]. Surprisingly, these mice developed a highly significant protective immunity after vaccination with ts-4. In order to understand how these CD8+ deficient animals are protected, we examined their spleen cell populations after vaccination. CD8+ counts, as expected, were drastically reduced while CD4+ numbers were largely unchanged. However, an enormous increase in a non-B, non-T cell population was observed. These cells stained positively with antibody to the NK cell antigen NK1.1. Moreover, when vaccinated β-2 microglobulin mice were treated with antibodies against asialoGM$_1$ (an NK cell surface determinant distinct from NK1.1.), protective immunity was ablated and the NK1.1 splenic population was markedly reduced. When stimulated with parasite antigen, spleen cells from vaccinated deficient mice produced levels of IFN-γ comparable to those produced by spleen cells from vaccinated non-deficient mice. Nevertheless, almost all of this cytokine was shown to be derived from a non-T cell population removed by *in vivo* anti-asialoGM$_1$ antibody treatment. The above findings argue that NK cells can compensate for CD8+ lymphocytes as effector cells of immunity to toxoplasma. They appear to do so by producing IFN-γ but may also function as cytolytic cells (Figure 1).

In order to understand how *T.gondii* might trigger NK cells, we have been studying the interaction of the parasite with NK enriched spleen cells from *scid* mice [Bancroft *et al* 1991]. These non-B, non-T populations respond to small numbers of tachyzoites or soluble tachyzoite antigens by producing high levels of IFN-γ. The molecules in the parasite which stimulate the response are heat-labile. IFN-γ production by *scid* spleen cells is dependent on NK cells, an adherent cell (co-stimulatory) population, and on TNF-α. However, TNF-α alone or TNF-α plus *T.gondii* is insufficient to trigger a cytokine response from purified NK cells. Experiments using supernatants from macrophages cultured with parasite extracts suggest that some other parasite stimulated factor or monokine ("Factor 'x'") is required (Figure 2). The requirement for co-stimulation can be partially overcome by the addition of IL-2 to the cultures suggesting that under these conditions NK cells can be directly stimulated by parasite products (Figure 2). That T-independent triggering of NK cells can act as an initial host defence against the parasite is supported by experiments in which *scid* mice were shown to become more susceptible to primary infection (as indicated by increased mortality) as a consequence of treatment with either anti-IFN-γ or anti-asialoGM$_1$ antibodies.

In conclusion, these studies suggest that resistance against *Toxoplasma gondii* involves a complicated interplay between CD4+, CD8+ T lymphocytes and NK cells in which each cell population is capable of partly or completely

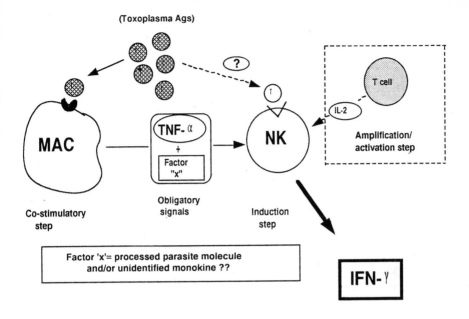

Figure 2. Proposed pathway for T-independent triggering of IFN-γ from NK
cells by *Toxoplasma gondii*.

compensating for the function of the other (Figure 1). The key property which
the three cells share is the ability to produce IFN-γ, a crucial mediator of
resistance against the parasite. Nevertheless, we believe (see above) that in
non-immunodeficient hosts, the major function of CD4+ cells is to provide
help for CD8+ (and perhaps NK) cells which then function as IFN-γ
producers and/or cytolytic cells (Figure 1). NK cells, in addition to providing
an initial T-independent defence barrier, could through their production of IFN-
γ bias the subsequent CD4+ response toward the expansion of Th1 cells since
Th2 cell proliferation is known to be suppressed by that cytokine. The
elucidation of the functional role of these different cellular interactions as well

as the parasite molecules which stimulate them is a challenging and highly relevant area for future research.

REFERENCES

Bancroft GJ, Schreiber RD, Unanue ER [1991] Natural immunity: a T-cell-independent pathway of macrophage activation, defined in the *scid* mouse. Immunol Rev 124: 5-24.

Gazzinelli RT, Hakim FT, Hieny S, Shearer GM, Sher A [1991] Synergistic role of CD4+ and CD8+ T lymphocytes in IFN-γ production and protective immunity induced by an attenuated *Toxoplasma gondii* vaccine. J Immunol 146: 286-292.

Gazzinelli RT, Xu Y, Hieny S, Cheever A, Sher A [1992] Simulataneous depletion of CD4+ and CD8+ T lymphocytes is required to re-activate chronic infection with *Toxoplasma gondii*. J. Immunol, in press.

Hakim FT, Gazzinelli RT, Denkers E, Hieny S, Shearer GM, Sher A [1991] CD8+ T cells from mice vaccinated against *Toxoplasma gondii* are cytotoxic for parasite-infected or antigen-pulsed host cells. J Immunol 147: 2310-2316.

Koller BH, Marrack P, Kappler JW, Smithies O [1990] Normal development of mice deficient in β-2 microglobulin, MHC class I proteins, and CD8+ T cells. Science 248: 1227-1230.

Subauste CS, Koniaris AH, Remington JS [1991] Murine CD8+ cytotoxic T lymphocytes lyse *Toxoplasma gondii*-infected cells. J Immunol 147: 3955-3959.

Suzuki Y, Orellana MA, Schreiber RD, Remington JS [1988] Interferon-γ: The major mediator of resistance against *Toxoplasma gondii*. Science 240: 516-518.

HUMAN T-CELL CLONES AS TOOLS TO IDENTIFY PROTECTIVE ANTIGENS OF *TOXOPLASMA GONDII*

P. Hérion[1,3] and R Saavedra[2]
[1]Innogenetics N.V.
Industriepark Zwijnaarde, 7
B-9052 Ghent
Belgium

Introduction

Many *in vitro* and *in vivo* observations indicate that cell-mediated immunity plays an essential role in protection of the host against toxoplasmosis. In the mouse experimental model, it has recently been shown that both CD4+ and CD8$^+$ lymphocytes are important in controlling acute infection and preventing reactivation of chronic toxoplasmosis [Suzuki and Remington, 1988; Araujo, 1991; Gassinelli et al, 1991; Gazzinelli et al 1992]. The exact mechanism by which these T-cell subsets confer protection has not yet been fully elucidated, but two lymphokines (IL-2 and IFN-γ) produced by these T-cells have been demonstrated to have a protective activity [Sharma et al., 1985]; Suzuki et al., 1988; Suzuki and Remington, 1990; Suzuki et al. 1990; Gazzinelli et al., 1991]. Parasite-specific T-cell clones (TCC) derived from naturally infected and immune individuals offer an ingenious way to dissect the cell-mediated immune response and to identify the parasite antigens which induce protective effector mechanisms. Such antigens should thus be considered as subunit vaccine candidates.

---

[2] Departamento de Immunologia, Instituto de Investigaciones Biomédicas, Universidad Nacional Autonoma de Mexico, AP 70228 Ciudad Universitaria 04510 Mexico DF, Mexico.
[3] Present address: see [2].

NATO ASI Series, Vol. H 78
Toxoplasmosis
Edited by Judith E. Smith
© Springer-Verlag Berlin Heidelberg 1993

Isolation and characterization of *T. gondii*-specific human T-cell clones

T. gondii-specific TCC were derived from a naturally infected/immune blood donor by *in vitro* stimulation of peripheral blood lymphocytes with a crude preparation of soluble tachyzoite antigens named F3 (supernatant of a tachyzoite sonicate after centrifugation at 100,000 g), and limiting dilution cloning. A panel of 15 clones, whose specificity for *T. gondii* was demonstrated by proliferation assay, was further characterized with respect to phenotype and production of IL-2 and IFN-γ after antigenic stimulation (Table 1).

Table 1. *Toxoplasma gondii*-reactive human T-cell clones: phenotype and lymphokine production.

Clone	Phenotype	IFN- (IU/ml)		L-2 (u/ml)
		F3	F3 + IL-2	F3
1G5	CD4	11	30	<0.16
2G4	CD4	65	100	<0.16
2E3	CD4	10	80	<0.16
2G8	CD4	73	95	2.0
29B	CD4	10	48	<0.16
210	CD4	35	55	0.2
26	CD4	23	52	<0.16
216	CD4	18	36	<0.16
21	CD4	8	35	<0.26
31	CD4	80	105	1.8
32	CD4	1400	1300	15
35	CD4	190	250	0.9
27	CD4	5	21	<0.16
34	CD4	47	115	<0.16
215	CD8	6	32	<0.16
None (APC only)		5	20	<0.16

T cells were stimulated with F3 in the presence of irradiated autologous peripheral blood mononuclear cells as antigen-presenting cells (APC), with or without addition of exogenous IL-2 (10 u/ml). IL-2 was determined in the supernatant using the bioassay described by Gillis et al.(1978). IFN-γ was determined by an immunoradiometric assay. Control cultures were carried out in parallel without F3; in the supernatant of these cultures IL-2 concentration was always <0.16 u/ml and IFN-γ concentration was always <5 IU/ml (adapted from Saavedra and Hérion (1991).

It is noteworthy that the majority of the clones (14/15) belong to the CD4 subset and only one clone belongs to the CD8 subset. The predominance of the CD4 subset does not seem to result from a selection caused by the *in vitro* culture conditions but most probably reflects the asymptomatic chronic infection status of the donor [Saavedra and Hérion, 1991]. Conversely, parasite-specific CD8[+] clones have been isolated with a higher frequency from donors with acute symptomatic infection [Sklenar et al., 1986; Yano et al., 1989]. Examination of the lymphokine production levels indicates a high heterogeneity of the TCC. Only five of the clones produced detectable levels of IL-2 whereas nine clones produced significant amounts of IFN-γ. In some cases, and particularly for the CD8[+] clone, IFN-γ production was dependent on the presence of exogenous IL-2.

As clone 32 produced a remarkably high level of both lymphokines, it was considered as potentially protective and further characterized. Blocking experiments with monoclonal antibodies directed against class I and class II HLA molecules and proliferation assays using a panel of HLA-typed B-lymphoblastoid cell lines as antigen-presenting cells indicated that antigen recognition by TCC 32 was restricted by the DPw4 molecule [Saavedra et al., 1991]. Since this allele is found at a high frequency in the population (40-70% among Caucasians, 10% among Japanese), a large fraction thereof is genetically competent to mount an immune response to the TCC 32-defined epitope.

Cloning and characterization of a potentially protective antigen

Molecular identification of the antigen defined by TCC 32 was achieved by constructing a cDNA library in the cloning/expression vector lambda gt11, screening this library with a pool of immune human sera, and testing the ability of the selected recombinant antigens to induce proliferation of TCC 32. One of 44 recombinant clones tested (clone Tg 34) produced an antigen which specifically stimulated TCC 32 proliferation [Saavedra et al., 1991].

The nucleotide sequence of this cDNA clone was determined and displays no homology with other previously described *T. gondii* genes. It contains a single long open reading frame with a coding capacity for a polypeptide of calculated molecular mass 61.5 kDa. Isolation and characterization by restriction analysis of a genomic clone containing this gene also indicated the absence of intron [Hérion, unpublished results]. Using antibodies specific for the recombinant form of this antigen, it was shown that the mature natural antigen present in the parasite has an apparent MW of 54 kDa suggesting a possible processing from a precursor form [Saavedra et al. 1991].

The predicted protein sequence contains a stretch of hydrophobic amino acids at its amino terminus presumably corresponding to a signal sequence; the presence of a second hydrophobic region spanning from residue 464 to 485 and predicted as transmembranous suggests that this antigen is membrane-associated. Immunofluorescence and immunoelectronmicroscopy subcellular localization studies carried out with antibodies raised against a recombinant form of the antigen showed that this antigen is localized in the rhoptries, one of the organelles of the apical complex of the zoite involved in host cell invasion. More precisely, the Tg34-encoded antigen was shown to be the previously termed ROP 2 rhoptry protein since the recombinant product reacted specifically with mAb 2F8 and 2D1 used to define this antigen (Hérion et al., submitted).

ROP 2 is known to be expressed in the three stages of the *T. gondii* life cycle (tachyzoite, bradyzoite, and sporozoite) [Sadak et al., 1988]. The T-cell epitope defined by TCC 32 on this antigen was also shown to be conserved among strains of various host and geographical origins and of different phenotypes (the virulent RH strain isolated from a patient in the U.S., the virulent Wiktor strain isolated from a rabbit in Zaïre and the non-virulent, cyst-forming Gangji strain isolated from a patient in Belgium) [Saavedra et al., 1991]. Moreover, antibodies against a recombinant form of this protein were detected in the serum of most individuals (83%) with serologically proven acute or chronic toxoplasmosis as well as in the serum of all mice experimentally infected with eleven independent *T. gondii* isolates [Van Gelder et al., submitted]. The high degree of conservation of this antigen suggests that it could have an essential function (probably in the host cell invasion process) and also strengthens its value as vaccine candidate.

Acknowledgements

We thank F. de Meuter, Rogelio Hernanswz-Pando, P. Van Gelder, J.L. Decourt, and J.F. Dubremetz for their collaboration.

References

Araujo F.G. [1991] Depletion of L3T4$^+$ (CD4$^+$) T lymphocytes prevents development of resistance to *Toxoplasma   gondii* in mice. Infect Immun 59 : 1614-1619.

Gazzinelli R.T., Hakim F.T., Hieny S., Shearer G.M., and Sher A [1991] Synergistic role of CD4$^+$ and CD8$^+$ T lymphocytes in IFN-γ production and protective immunity induced by an attenuated *Toxoplasma   gondii* vaccine. J. Immunol 146 : 286-292.

Gazzinelli R.T., Xu Y., Hieny S., Cheever A., and Sher A [1992] Simultaneous depletion of CD4$^+$ and CD8$^+$ lymphocytes is required to re-activate chronic infection with *Toxoplasma   gondii*. J. Immunol (in press).

Gillis S., Ferm M.M., Ou W and Smith K.A. [1978] T cell growth factor: parameters of production and a quantitative microassay for activity. J. Immunol 120: 2027-2032.

Hérion P., Hernandex-Pando R., Dubremetz J.F., and Saavedra R. The potentially protective 54-kDa antigen of *Toxoplasma   gondii* is the rhoptry protein ROP 2. Submitted for publication.

Saavedra R and Hérion P [1991] Human T-cell clones against *Toxoplasma gondii* : production of interferon-γ, interleukin- 2, and strain cross-reactivity. Parasitol Res 77: 739-385.

Saavedra R., De Meuter F., Decourt J.L. and Hérion P [1991] Human T cell clone identifies a potentially protective 54-kDa protein antigen of *Toxoplasma   gondii* cloned and expressed in *Escherichia   coli*. J. Immunol 147: 1975-1982.

Sadak   A., Taghy   Z.,   Fortier   B   and   Dubremetz   J.F.   [1988] Characterization of a family of rhoptry proteins of *Toxoplasma   gondii*. Mol Biochem Parasitol 29: 202-211.

Sharma S.D., Hofflin J.M. and Remington J.S. [1985] In vivo recombinant interleukin 2 administration enhances survival against a lethal challenge with Toxoplasma gondii. J Immunol 135: 4140-4163.

Sklenar I., Jones T.C., Alkan S. and Erb P [1986] Association of symptomatic human infection with *Toxoplasma   gondii* with imbalance of monocytes and antigen-specific T cell subsets. J Infect Dis 153: 315-324.

Suzuki Y and Remington J.S. [1988] Dual regulation of resistance against *Toxoplasma gondii* infection by Lyt-2$^+$ and Lyt-1$^+$, L3T4$^+$ T cells in mice. J. Immunol 140: 3943-3946.

Suzuki Y., Orellana M.A., Schreiber R.D., and Remington J.S. [1988] Interferon-γ *Toxoplasma gondii*. Science 240: 516-518.

Suzuki Y and Remington J.S. [1990] The effect of anti-IFN-γ antibody on the protective effect of Lyt2$^+$ immune T cells against toxoplasmosis in mice. J. Immunol 144: 1954-1956.

Suzuki Y., Conley F.K. and Remington, J.S. [1990] Treatment of toxoplasmic encephalitis in mice with recombinant gamma interferon. Infect Immun 58: 3050-3055.

Van Gelder P., Bosman F., De Meuter F., Van Heuverswyn H and Hérion P. Serodiagnosis of toxoplasmosis using a recombinant form of the 54-kDa rhoptry antigen expressed in *Escherichia coli*. Submitted for publication.

Yano A., Aosai F., Ohta M., Hasekura H., Sugane K. and Hayashi S [1989] Antigen presentation by *Toxoplasma gondii* - infected cells to CD4$^+$ proliferative T cells and CD8$^+$ cytotoxic cells. J Parasitol 75: 411-416.

PROTECTION OF MICE AND NUDE RATS AGAINST TOXOPLASMOSIS BY AN OCTAMERIC CONSTRUCT OF THE P30 48-67 PEPTIDE.

F. Darcy[1,2], P. Maes[3], H. Gras-Masse[3], I. Godard[1], M. Bossus[3], C. Auriault[1], D. Deslée[1], M. F. Cesbron[1], A. Tartar[3], and A. Capron[1].
[1]Centre d'Immunologie et de Biologie Parasitaire
INSERM U167 - CNRS 624
Institut Pasteur de Lille
1 rue du Pr. Calmette
59019 Lille Cedex
France

The sequence of the first 20 NH2-terminus residues of P30 were obtained from this major surface antigen of *T. gondii* purified by HPLC. A synthetic peptide (P30 48-67) has been prepared both in linear form and as an octameric construction. Immunization of mice and rats with the P30 48-67 octamer in the presence of IFA induces high levels of IgG antibodies which recognize both the monomeric and the octameric peptides in ELISA, and P30 in Western blots of NP40-extracted tachyzoite antigens. Since these sera are negative in immunofluorescence assays with whole tachyzoites, it seems that IgG antibodies induced by P30 48-67 octamer, although recognizing the denatured structure, are unable to recognize the native protein. The protective effect of both constructs has been studied in mice and Nude rats. Whereas immunization of mice with the monomeric peptide does not confer any protection against oral infection with 1200 cysts of *T. gondii* 76K strain (mortality within 11 days), 40% of mice immunized with the octameric construct survived up to 75 days after infection. Nude rats were passively transferred with 5×10^4 T lymphocytes from P30 48-67 octamer-immunized Fischer rats before infection with 5×10^4 RH strain tachyzoites. When compared to Nude rats transferred with control T lymphocytes, they presented an almost two-fold increase in their mean survival time and raised an intense IgG antibody response against P30. This shows that immunization with P30 48-67 MAP also induces an efficient T cell immune response. The present work confirms the recently demonstrated role of P30 in protective immunity and shows the interest of peptide octameric constructions as inducers of partially protective immune responses in toxoplasmosis, as already demonstrated in schistosomiasis.

---

[2]Present address : INSERM U298, CHRU, 49033 Angers Cedex 01, France
[3]Laboratoire de Chimie des Biomolécules, URA CNRS 1309, Institut Pasteur de Lille, France

NATO ASI Series, Vol. H 78
Toxoplasmosis
Edited by Judith E. Smith
© Springer-Verlag Berlin Heidelberg 1993

INTRODUCTION

Our laboratory had been interested for years in P30 (SAG1), the major surface antigen of *Toxoplasma gondii* tachyzoites, mostly due to its diagnostic interest. Indeed, we have developed IgM (Santoro et al., 1985) and IgA (Decoster et al., 1988) immunocapture tests using the TG54 monoclonal antibody directed against P30. In addition, the observation that the passive transfer of the TG54 monoclonal antibody to nude rats significantly prolonged their survival after infection with the highly virulent *T. gondii* RH strain (Santoro et al., 1987) suggested protective potentialities for this major antigen. After purification of P30 by HPLC, we obtained a partial amino-acid sequence, which was later found to be identical to residues 48-67 of the predicted amino-acid sequence deduced from a cDNA clone (Burg et al., 1988). However, this 20 amino-acid sequence was the only information available to us at this time. Considering the promising results obtained in our laboratory in the case of a peptide octameric construct of the P28 protein of S. Mansoni (Wolowczuk et al., 1991), we have constructed the P30 48-67 peptide both in monomeric and in octameric forms.

The immunogenicity of these synthetic peptides and their protective potentialities against toxoplasmosis were then explored in mice and rats.

RESULTS

Selection of the peptide constructs

P30 was isolated in a pure form from tachyzoite antigens solubilized with NP40 by reversed phase HPLC. The sequence of the first twenty NH_2 - terminus residues, determined by gas-phase microsequencing, was as follows :

Ser-Asp-Pro-Pro-Leu-Val-Ala-Asn-Gln-Val-Val-Thr-Cys-Pro-Asp-Lys-Lys-Ser-Thr-Ala

Considering the presence in this region of a Pro - Pro bond which , due to its slow isomerization rate, is likely to generate a stable spatial organization suitable to be reproduced by a short peptide, we decided to explore the immunogenicity of synthetic constructs. In addition to this P30 48-67 (numbering according to Burg et al., 1988) linear peptide, we also prepared an octameric form of P30 48-67 based on the multiple antigenic peptide method proposed by Tam (1988). This octameric peptide consisted in a branched core of lysine residues on which eight identical copies of the peptide are linked (Fig.1).

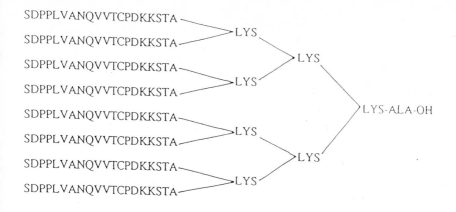

Fig. 1 : Structure of the octameric construction of P30 48-67 peptide

The thiol group of cystein was protected by a permanent acetamidomethyl group in order to avoid the uncontrolled formation of disulfide bonds between the peptide chains.

In order to detect possible non specific reactions which could be generated by the polylysine core, a second construct bearing eight copies of an irrelevant peptide (sequence : Ala - Lys - Glu - Pro - Ser - Phe - Asn - Gly - Thr - Val - Asp - Leu) was also prepared.

Protection of mice by immunization with the P30 48-67 peptide

Female Swiss mice were subcutaneously (s.c.) immunized on days 42, 35, 27 and 7 (before infection) with 25 ug of P30 48-67 monomeric or octameric peptide constructs, or of the irrelevant octamer in the presence of incomplete Freund's adjuvant (IFA). They were then orally infected with 1200 cysts of *T. gondii* 76K strain (Laugier and Quilici, 1970). Data obtained from three different experiments showed that 75 days after infection, 10 out of 27 mice immunized with the P30 48-67 octameric construct survived compared with 3 out of 31 mice immunized with the irrelevant octamer, this is highly significant according to the Chi^2 test (p<0.01).

Protection of Nude rats by passive transfer of P30 48-67 octamer - specific T cells.

Male Fischer rats were s. c. immunized on days 42, 35, 24 and 7 (before collection of lymphocytes) with 50 μg of P30 48-67 octamer or with the irrevelant octameric construct in the presence of IFA. Inguinal, periaortic and mesenteric lymph nodes were aseptically harvested and T cells were separated through a nylon wool column. These preparations contained 90 to 95% T cells (W3/13[+]) and 0% Bcells (OX 12[+]). Nude rats were intravenously injected with 5×10^4 T cells specific for the P30 or irrelevant octameric constructs, one day before intraperitoneal infection with 5×10^4 RH strain tachyzoites.

While the 2 groups of rats showed an equal mortality, the Nude rats having received P30 48-67 octamer-specific T lymphocytes demonstrated an almost two-fold increase in their mean survival time (29.8 days instead of 17 days), that is significant according to the Student's test (p<0.01).

Results from another experiment were similar. The mean time-to-death of the Nude rats transferred with P30 48-67 octamer-specific T lymphocytes was 1.8 fold that observed in the control group.

Antibody response of mice and rats immunized with P30 48-67 peptides.

Sera were tested in ELISA to check whether immunization of mice and Fischer rats with P30 48-67 peptides induced antibodies directed against these peptides. In sera from mice immunized either with the P30 48-67 linear peptide or with the P30 48-67 octamer, a high optical density (>2.5) was observed towards both forms of the parent peptide. Sera from Fischer rats immunized with P30 48-67 octamer also showed a high level of IgG antibodies directed against P30 48-67 peptides in both forms, when compared to sera from rats immunized with the irrelevant octameric construct.

Western blotting, using NP40-extracted *T. gondii* antigens, revealed a strong antibody response directed against P30 in sera from mice and Fischer rats immunized with P30 48-67 octamer. In contrast, the sera from mice immunized with P30 48-67 monomer only faintly reacted with P30 in Western blot.

Interestingly, the same sera from mice and rats immunized with P30 48-67 octamer were negative in immunofluorescence assay against tachyzoites.

Helper activity of T cells from donor Fischer rats immunized with the P30 48-67 octameric peptide.

In order to analyze the helper activity of P30 48-67 octamer - specific T cells, 5 x 10^4 T cells, directly recovered from immunized Fischer rats, were transferred into four Nude rats one day before infection with 5 x 10^4 RH strain tachyzoites. The sera from these Nude rats were collected every week from Day 13 after infection, then tested by Western blotting .

Twenty days post infection, IgG antibodies from 2 out of 4 Nude rats recognized a band at 30 kDa. From Day 27 onwards, IgG from 3 out of 4 rats intensely recognized P30. These results demonstrate that the adoptive transfer of only 5 x 10^4 specific T lymphocytes to the Nude rats induces the production of antibodies directed against the P30 antigen. The fact that 1 out the 4 protected rats did not present any IgG response suggests that antibodies were not necessary for the conferred protection.

DISCUSSION

The interest of P30 peptides in protection against toxoplasmosis has been very recently strengthened by two reports which demonstrated that immunization with P30, either incorporated into liposomes (Bülow and Boothroyd, 1991) or in the presence of Quil A (Khan et al., 1991) confers a nearly 100% protection to mice infected with moderately virulent strains of T. Gondii .

The present work evidences the high immunogenicity of the P30 48-67 peptide in the form of an octameric construct, even in the absence of any carrier protein.

Immunization with P30 48-67 octamer induces, in both mice and rats, a high level of IgG antibodies which recognize in ELISA both the monomeric and the octameric form of the parent peptide. These antibodies strongly react against P30 in immunoblots but do not recognize the native surface antigen in immunofluorescence assays. It thus seems likely that the antibodies induced by immunizations with P30 48-67 synthetic peptides are directed towards linear epitopes present either in the peptides themselves or in P30 after SDS-denaturation, but are unable to recognize the conformational epitopes exposed at the parasite surface.

The protective role of the two forms of the P30 48-67 peptide has been evaluated in two experimental models, mice and Nude rats. The Nude rat model was chosen because, while immunocompetent rats are resistant to toxoplasmosis

(Chinchilla et al., 1982), Nude rats do not survive an infection with 10^3 RH strain tachyzoites . Their protection can be restored by the passive transfer of 5 x 10^6 non immune T cells (Santoro et al., 1987). We show here that the adoptive transfer of only 5 x 10^4 specific T cells from Fischer rats immunized with P30 48-67 octamer significantly prolonges the survival of these athymic rats, since a nearly 2 fold increase of their time-to-death after infection with 5 x 10^4 RH strain tachyzoites was observed. This demonstrates that, besides the B cell response reported above, immunization with the P30 48-67 octameric construct also induces an efficient T cell immune response.

In addition, the data presented here demonstrate that the T cell epitope present in the P30 48-67 peptide elicits *in vivo* functional T cells that help the production of IgG antibodies directed against P30 by the majority of the transferred, then infected, Nude rats. Since one rat was protected despite the lack of production of anti-P30 antibodies, it seems likely that the P30 48-67 octamer- induced T cells could also be involved in antibody-independent cellular effector mechanisms.They could act through the production of lymphokines in particular interferon γ, the major mediator of resistance against mouse toxoplasmosis (Suzuki et al., 1988 ; Suzuki and Remington, 1990) although we have recently shown that IFNγ exerts a smaller protective effect against Nude rat toxoplasmosis (Benedetto et al., 1991). Another hypothesis is the induction of cytotoxic T lymphocytes (CTL) since Khan et al. (1988) have described that P30 induces in mice CTL that are directly cytotoxic for extracellular parasites. Most of the data from recent investigations of *in vivo* experimental models point to a major role of CD8$^+$ T cells in host resistance to *T. Gondii*. Indeed, the CD8$^+$ T cells from mice vaccinated either with the TS-4 mutant of *T. Gondii* (Gazzinelli et al., 1991 ; Hakim et al., 1991 ; Subauste et al., 1991) or with P30 (Kasper et al., 1992) are cytotoxic for parasite-infected cells. It would be of interest to further investigate whether, within the amino-acid sequence of P30, the 48-67 peptide presented as an octameric construction could elicit, after s.c. immunization, CD8$^+$T lymphocytes directly cytotoxic for the tachyzoites and the *Toxoplasma*-infected cells.

The protective potentialities of P30 48-67 octamer have also been explored in the mouse model by direct immunization. The oral infection of Swiss mice with 1200 cysts of *T. Gondii* 76K strain leads to a fairly constant level of mortality (Darcy et al., 1992). In this model, immunization with the P30 48-67 octameric construct induced a highly significant degree of protection (about 40%) whereas the P30 48-67 monomeric peptide did not improve mouse survival. It is of interest to note that in these non protected mice immunized with the P30 48-67 monomer,

IgG antibodies only faintly reacted with P30 in Western blots. In addition, and since in mouse toxoplasmosis cell-mediated immunity is predominant, it is likely that mouse immunization with P30 48-67 monomeric peptide does not stimulate cellular immunity as efficiently as does the octameric construct.

Our results represent, to our knowledge, the first example of a partial, but significant protection obtained against *T. Gondii* infection by immunizing with a molecule as small as a construct derived from a 20 amino-acid peptide. This suggests, as already reported in schistosomiasis (Wolowczuk et al., 1991), the potential interest of peptide octameric constructions as subunit vaccines. Since it is likely that an efficient strategy of vaccination against toxoplasmosis will only be obtained by the combination of various parasite antigenic structures, it is worth investigating the protective potentialities of similar constructs from other peptides, derived for instance from P30 (SAG1), P23 (GRA1, Cesbron-Delauw et al., 1989) in which T cell epitopes have been identified (Duquesne et al., 1991) or GP28.5 (GRA2, Mercier et al., in preparation). In addition, the degree of protection afforded by the P30 48-67 octameric construct might likely be improved through modifications of the immunization protocols, such as oral route of administration, incorporation into liposomes and iscoms, and testing a range of adjuvants such as Quil A and cholera toxin for instance.

ACKNOWLEDGEMENTS

We thank Mrs Martine Larfouilloux and Léna Manoukian for their assistance in the preparation of this manuscript.

REFERENCES

Benedetto N, C Auriault, F Darcy, D Lando, H Watier, and A Capron. (1991). Effect of IFNγ and IL2 treatments in mouse and nude rate infections with *Toxoplasma gondii*. Eur. Cytokine Net. 2 : 107.

Bülow R, and JC Boothroyd . (1991). Protection of mice from fatal *Toxoplasma gondii* infection by immunization with P30 antigen in liposomes. J. Immunol. 147 : 3496.

Burg JL, D Perelman, LH Kasper, PL Ware, and JC Boothroyd. (1988). Molecular analysis of the gene encoding the major surface antigen of *Toxoplasma gondii*. J. Immunol. 141 : 3584.

Cesbron-Delauw MF, B Guy, G Torpier, RJ Pierce, G. Lenzen, JY Cesbron, H Charif, P Lepage, F Darcy, JP Lecocq, and A Capron. (1989). Molecular characterization of a 23kDa major antigen secreted by *Toxoplasma gondii*. Proc. Natl. Acad. Sci. USA; 86 : 7537.

Chinchilla M, OM Guerrero, and E Solano. (1982). Lack of multiplication of *Toxoplasma* in macrophages of rats *in vitro*. J. Parasitol. 68 : 952.

Darcy F, G Torpier, MF Cesbron-Delauw, A Decoster, and A Capron. (1992). Diagnostic et prévention de la toxoplasmose : nouvelles approches et perspectives. Gynecol. Internat. 1 : 48.

Decoster A, F Darcy, A Caron, and A Capron. (1988). IgA antibodies against P30 as markers of congenital and acute toxoplasmosis. Lancet ii : 1104.

Duquesne V, C Auriault, H Gras-Masse, C Boutillon, F Darcy, MF Cesbron-Delauw, A Tartar, and A Capron. (1991). Identification of T cell epitopes within a 23-kD antigen (P24) of *Toxoplasma gondii*. Clin. Exp. Immunol. 84 : 527.

Gazzinelli RT, FT Hakim, F Hieny, GM Shearer, and A Sher. (1991). Synergistic role of CD4$^+$ and CD8$^+$ T-lymphocytes in IFN-γ production and protective immunity induced by an attenuated *Toxoplasma gondii* vaccine. J. Immunol. 146 : 286.

Hakim FT, RT Gazzinelli, E Denkers, S Hieny, GM Shearer, and A Sher. (1991). CD8$^+$ T cells from mice vaccinated against *Toxoplasma gondii* are cytotoxic for parasite-infected or antigen-pulsed host cells. J. Immunol. 147-2310.

Kasper LH, IA Khan, KH Ely, R Buelow, and JC Boothroyd. (1992). Antigen-specific (P30) mouse CD8$^+$ T cells are cytotoxic against *Toxoplasma gondii*-infected peritoneal macrophages. J. Immunol. 148-1493.

Khan IA, KH Ely, and LH Kasper. (1991). A purified parasite antigen (P30) mediates CD8$^+$ T cell immunity against fatal *Toxoplasma gondii* infection in mice. J. Immunol. 147 : 3501.

Khan IA, KA Smith, and LH Kasper. (1988). Induction of antigen-specific parasiticidal cytotoxic T cell splenocytes by a major membrane protein (P30) of *Toxoplasma gondii*. J. Immunol. 141 : 3600.

Laugier M, and M Quilici. (1970). Intérêt expérimental d'une souche de toxoplasme peu pathogène pour la souris. Ann. Parasitol. Hum. Comp. 45 : 389.

Santoro F, D Afchain, R Pierce, JY Cesbron, G Ovlaque, and A Capron. (1985) Serodiagnosis of toxoplasma infection using a purified parasite protein (P30). Clin. Exp. Immunol. 62 : 262.

Santoro F, C Auriault, P Leite, F Darcy, and A Capron. (1987). Infection du rat athymique par *Toxoplasma gondii*. C.R. Acad. Sci. Ser III. 304 : 297.

Subauste C, AH Koniaris, and JS Remington. (1991). Murine CD8$^+$ cytotoxic lymphocytes lyse *Toxoplasma gondii*-infected cells. J. Immunol. 147 : 3955.

Suzuki Y, MA Orellana, RD Schreiber, and JS Remington. (1988). Interferon γ : the major mediator of resistance against *Toxoplasma gondii*. Science. 240 : 516.

Suzuki Y, and JS Remington. (1990). The effect of anti-IFNγ antibody on the protective effect of Lyt-2^+ immune T cells against toxoplasmosis in mice. J. Immunol. 144 : 1954.

Tam JP. (1988). Synthetic peptide vaccine design : synthesis and properties of a high-density multiple antigenic peptide system. Proc. Natl. Acad. Sci USA. 85 : 5409.

Wolowczuk I, C Auriault, M Bossus, D Boulanger, H Gras-Masse, C Mazingue, RJ Pierce, D Grezel, A Tartar, and A Capron. (1991). Antigenicity and immunogenicity of a multiple peptidic construction of the *Schistosoma mansoni* Sm-28GST antigen in rat, mouse and monkey. 1 Partial protection of Fischer rat after active immunisation. J. Immunol. 146 : 1987.

TOXOPLASMOSIS
VACCINES
DIAGNOSIS
&
CHEMOTHERAPY

SYNERGISTIC DRUG COMBINATIONS IN THE TREATMENT OF TOXOPLASMOSIS

Fausto G. Araujo, DVM, Ph.D.
Department of Immunology and Infectious Diseases
Research Institute, Palo Alto Medical Foundation
860 Bryant St., Palo Alto, CA, USA.

Abstract

In an attempt to improve the activity of azithromycin, clarithromycin or 566C80 against *Toxoplasma gondii*, combinations of these drugs with pyrimethamine or sulfadiazine were used for treatment of mice infected with the organism. Significant synergistic effect was noted when sub-curative doses of any of the examined drugs were combined with sub-curative doses of pyrimethamine or sulfadiazine. This was true even when the combination consisted of concentrations of each drug that, when used alone, afforded no protection against death. This observation was of interest since pyrimethamine and, particularly, sulfadiazine are major sources of untoward side-effects when used for treatment of toxoplasmosis in patients with AIDS. Therefore, a significant reduction in the dose of these drugs without lessening their effect against *T. gondii* may be useful.

Introduction

At present the treatment of choice for toxoplasmosis remains the synergistic combination of pyrimethamine and a sulfonamide [McCabe & Remington, 1990]. However, untoward side-effects that may require discontinuation of the therapy are relatively frequent when this combination is used to treat toxoplasmosis in immunocompromised individuals, particularly AIDS patients [Israelski et al, 1990]. Therefore, a considerable research effort is in progress to identify new therapeutic agents and new therapeutic combinations for treatment of toxoplasmosis, particularly toxoplasmic encephalitis. Recently, the azalide-macrolide antibiotics azithromycin and clarithromycin were found to be active against *T. gondii* [Araujo et al, 1991b]. In addition, the hydroxynaphthoquinone 566C80 (2-[trans-4-(clorophenyl)cyclohexyl)-3-hydroxy-1,4-naphthoquinone]) was shown to be remarkably active in protecting mice

NATO ASI Series, Vol. H 78
Toxoplasmosis
Edited by Judith E. Smith
© Springer-Verlag Berlin Heidelberg 1993

against death due to intraperitoneal or oral infection with various strains of the parasite [Araujo et al, 1992b]. Moreover, the numbers of *T. gondii* cysts in brains of chronically infected mice were reduced significantly by prolonged treatment of the animals with 566C80 [Araujo et al, 1991b].

The mechanisms of action of azalide-macrolide antibiotics and of 566C80 against *T. gondii* are still unclear. Macrolide antibiotics inhibit protein synthesis by binding to 50 S ribosomal subunits of sensitive microorganisms and hydroxynaphthoquinones are known to block pyrimidine synthesis by inhibiting the mitrochondrial electron transport chain in a number of parasitic protozoa [Araujo et al, 1992a, Vogel et al 1971]. These are, presumably, the mechanisms of activity of these antimicrobials against *T. gondii*. On the other hand, the mechanisms of action of pyrimethamine and sulfonamides against microorganisms, including *T. gondii*, involve interference with the synthesis of folic acid. Sulfonamides inhibit the utilization of para-aminobenzoic acid for the synthesis of dihydropteroic acid [Hammond et al, 1985] and pyrimethamine inhibits the reduction of dehydrofolate to tetrahydrofolate [Woods, 1962].

The apparently different modes of actions of pyrimethamine, sulfadiazine, macrolide antibiotics and hydroxynaphthoquinones against *T. gondii* suggested that combinations of these drugs may act synergistically in murine toxoplasmosis. This possibility was investigated *in vivo* using mice infected with *T. gondii* and treated with drug combinations.

Material and Methods

Drugs: Azithromycin (Pfizer Inc., Groton, CT, USA) was dissolved in a small volume of 95% ethanol and the concentrations for use were prepared in polyethylene glycol 200 (JT Baker Chem. Co., Phillipsburg, NJ, USA).Clarithromycin (Abbott Laboratories, Abbott Park, IL) was dissolved in phosphate buffered saline, pH, 6.8, sonicated before each dosage and given orally using a feeding needle.566C80 (Burroughs-Wellcome, Research Triangle Park, NC, USA) was dissolved in distilled water and the desired concentrations prepared in 0.25% carboxymethyl cellulose containing 0.05% Tween 20 and administered orally using a feeding needle. Pyrimethamine (Burroughs-Wellcome) was dissolved in carboxymethyl cellulose as above and also administered orally using a feeding needle. Sulfadiazine (Sigma Chemicals Co., St. Louis, MO, USA) was dissolved and administered in the drinking water.

Mice: Swiss-Webster or CBA/Ca females, weighing 20 g at the beginning of each experiment were used.

Toxoplasma gondii: Tachyzoites of the RH strain or tissue cysts of the C56 strain were used. Tachyzoites were obtained from the peritoneal cavities of previously infected mice [Araujo et al, 1991b]. In all experiments each mouse was infected i.p. with 2.5×10^3 organisms. This number of organisms represents at least 250 LD100. Tissue cysts were collected from brains of chromically infected mice [Araujo et al, 1991a] and each mouse was infected orally with 10 cysts which represent 10 LD100.
Statistical analysis of the data was done using the Chi square and the Mann-Whitney U tests.

Results
In repeated dose-response experiments in our laboratory, a single dose of azithromycin of 50 mg/kg/day, administered for 10 days beginning 24 hours after infection, did not confer any protection against death due to toxoplasmosis; a dose of 75 mg protected no more than 40% of infected mice. In addition, also in repeated experiments, a dose of sulfadiazine of 80 mg/L of drinking water was never found to be sufficient to protect mice infected with RH tachyzoites.   In contrast, these concentrations of azithromycin and sulfadiazine induced remarkable protection against death due to acute toxoplasmosis when used in combination. In at least two experiments 100% survival was noted in infected mice treated with 50 mg/kg/day of azithromycin in combination with 80 mg/L of sulfadiazine (Figure 1). Surviving mice were observed for 50 days following discontinuation of treatment and infection did not reactivate in any of them. One hundred percent of control mice treated with 50 mg/kg of azithromycin or 80 mg/L of sulfadiazine administered alone died by day 9 of infection (Figure 1). Further experiments revealed that a dose as low as 25 mg/kg of azithromycin combined with 80 mg/L of sulfadiazine protected 40% of infected mice (data not shown).
Similarly, the combination azithromycin-pyrimethamine was highly synergistic in murine toxoplasmosis. A dose of 50 mg/kg/day of azithromycin combined with a dose of 10 mg/kg/day of pyrimethamine protected 90% of infected mice (Figure 2).

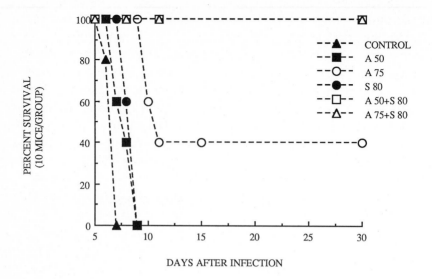

Figure 1. Activity of azithromycin (A) at the does of 50 or 75 mg/kg/day in combination with sulfadiazine (S) at the concentration of 80 mg/L of drinking water. Mice were infected with tachyzoites with tachyzoites and treatment was initiated 24 hours after infection and continued for 10 days.

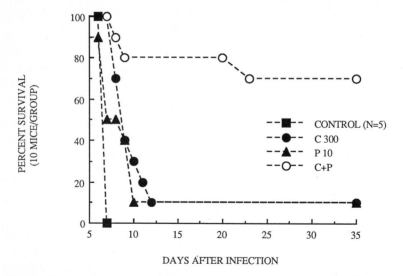

Figure 2. Activity of azithromycin (A) at the dose of 50 mg/kg/day in combination with pyrimethamine (P) at the dose of 10 mg/kg/day. Infection and treatment was as described in Fig. 1.

Previous experiments in our laboratory to determine the activity of clarithromycin in treatment of murine toxoplasmosis revealed varied results. However, in a number of experiments 10% to 30% of mice infected with lethal inocula of tachyzoites or tissue cysts and treated with a single daily dose of 300 mg/kg of clarithromycin administered for 10 days beginning 24 hours after infection survived for more than 30 days. Combination of this dose of clarithromycin with a dose of 10 mg/kg/day of pyrimethamine or a dose of 80 mg/L of sulfadiazine resulted in survival of 70% (Figure 3) or 60% (Figure 3) of the infected mice, respectively.

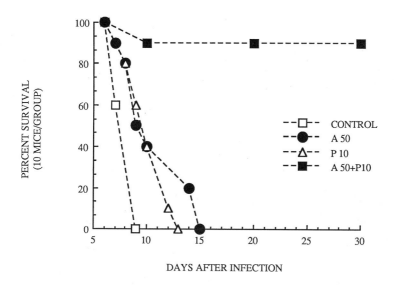

Figure 3. Activity of clarithromycin (C) at the dose of 300 mg/kg/day in combination with pyrimethamine (P) at the dose of 10 mg/kg/day. Infection and treatment was as descibed in Fig. 1.

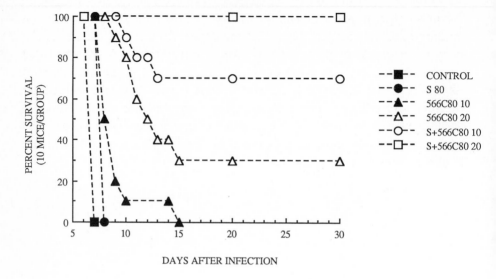

Figure 4. Activity of 566C80 at the doses of 10 or 20 mg/kg/day in combination with sulfadiazine (S) at the concentration of 80 mg/L of drinking water. Infection and treatment was as described in Fig. 1.

Previous results [Araujo et al, 1991a] revealed that a dose of 100 mg/kg/day of 566C80 administered for 10 days beginning up to 3 days after infection with RH tachyzoites protected 100% of mice against death. Infected mice treated with doses of 566C80 of 20 mg/kg or 10 mg/kg had approximately 30% survival or only a slight prolongation in time to death, respectively. When these low doses were combined with an ineffective dose of pyrimethamine (10 mg/kg/day) or sulfadiazine (80 mg/L) a remarkable synergistic effect was noted. Seventy and 100% of mice treated with combinations containing 10 or 20 mg/kg of 566C80 and 80 mg/L of sulfadiazine survived for up to 50 days when the experiment was terminated (Figure 4). A similar result was noted in mice infected with tissue cysts and treated with 566C80 in combination with sulfadiazine (Figure 5).

Although each of the antimicrobials examined in this work has been shown to be active in the treatment of murine toxoplasmosis when used alone, a variation in this activity has been demonstrated in mice infected with different strains of *T. gondii* [Araujo et al, 1991b, Araujo et al, 1991a], particularly when lower

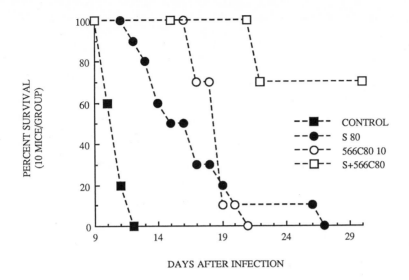

Figure 5. Activity of 566C80 at the dose of 10 mg/kg/day in combination with sulfadiazine (S) at the concentration of 80 mg/L of drinking water. Infection was with tissue cysts and treatment was initiated 3 days after infection and contrinued for 10 days.

than the optimal doses are used for treatment. Thus, an ample variation in the activity of 566C80 was noted when this drug was used at a dose of 20 mg/kg/day to treat mice infected with different strains of *T. gondii*. Of interest was that each one of the strains examined in this study, with the exception of the RH strain, was isolated from patients with AIDS and toxoplasmic encephalitis (Figure 6).

Discussion

The above results indicate that the combination of azithromycin, clarithromycin or 566C80 with sulfadiazine or pyrimethamine results in a remarkable synergistic effect in the treatment of murine toxoplasmosis. This was true even when the combination consisted of concentrations of each drug that, when used

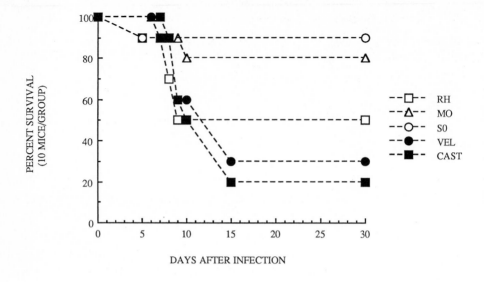

Figure 6. Activity of 566C80 at the dose of 20 mg/kg/day in mice infected with different strains of *T. gondii*. Strains MO, SO, VEL and CAST were from AIDS patients with toxoplasmic encephalitis. Infection was i.p. with equal numbers of tachyzoites and treatment was initiated 24 hours after infection and continued for 10 days.

alone, afforded no protection against death. This observation is of special interest because sulfadiazine is a frequent source of troublesome side-effects when used to treat AIDS patients with toxoplasmosis [Dannemann et al, 1992]. Therefore, a reduction in the dose of sulfadiazine used to treat these patients without lessening its effect may be helpful.

The problems posed by treatment of toxoplasmosis, particularly toxoplasmic encephalitis in patients with AIDS, have provided a powerful incentive and opportunity to improve therapy of this disease. New drugs lacking, or with diminished toxicity, as well as new therapeutic combinations which may allow shorter courses of therapy are urgently needed. The above results indicate that clinical trials using the combination of azithromycin, clarithromycin or 566C80 with a sulfonamide or with pyrimethamine for treatment of toxoplasmosis in AIDS patients is justified.

As it was reported with azithromycin [Araujo et al, 1991b], clarithromycin [Araujo et al, 1992c] and 566C80 [Araujo et al, 1992d] and Figure 5), significant variation in the activity of each one of these drugs occurs when they are used to treat mice infected with different strains of *T. gondii*. The implications that this observation may have for therapy of toxoplasmosis, particularly in AIDS patients with toxoplasmic encephalitis, is unclear at this moment. It is clear, however, that further work to define the significance and the mechanisms of strain variation in response to therapeutic agents is urgently needed.

Acknowledgements

The excellent technical expertise of T. Lin was appreciated. This work was supported by the United States Public Health Service grant AI30230 from the National Institutes of Health.

References

Araujo F.G., Huskinson J., and Remington J.S. [1991a] Remarkable *in vitro* and *in vivo* activities of the hydroxynaphthoquinone 566C80 against tachyzoites and cysts of *Toxoplasma gondii*. Antimicrob Agents and Chemother 35: 293-299.

Araujo F.G., Shepard R.M., and Remington J.S. [1991b] *In vivo* activity of the macrolide antibiotics azithromycin, roxithromycin and spiramycin against *Toxoplasma gondii*. Eur J Clin Microbiol Infect Dis 10: 519-524.

Araujo F.G., Huskinson-Mark J., Gutteridge W.E., Remington J.S. [1992a] *In vitro* and *in vivo* activities of the hydroxynaphthoquinone 566C80 against the cyst form of *Toxoplasma gondii*. Antimicrob Agents and Chemother 36: 326-330.

Araujo F.G., Prokocimer P. and Remington J.S. [1992b] Clarithromycin-minocycline is synergistic in a murine model of toxoplasmosis. J Infect Dis 165: 788.

Araujo F.G., Prokocimer Ph., Remington J.S. [1992c] Activity of clarithromycin in 'Murine models of toxoplasmosis'. Program and Abstracts of the 8th Mediterranean Congress of Chemotherapy. Athens, Greece, May 24-29, Abstract 728 pp 550.

Hammond D.J., Burchell J.R. and Pudney M. [1985] Inhibition of pyrimidine biosynthesis de novo in *Plasmodium falciparum* by 2-(4-t-butylcyclohexyl)-3-hydroxy-1,4-naphthoquinone *in vitro*. Mol Biochem Parasitol 14: 97-109.

Israelski D.M., Dannemann B.R. and Remington J.S. [1990] Toxoplasmosis in patients with AIDS. In 'The medical management of AIDS', ed. M.A. Sande and P.A. Volberding, Philadelphia: W.B. Saunders 241-264.

McCabe R.E. and Remington J.S. [1990] *Toxoplasma gondii*. In 'Third ed Principles and Practice of Infectious Diseases', ed G L Mandell, J Dauglas R G and J E Bennett London: Churchill Livingstone Inc 2090-2103.

Vogel Z., Vogel T., Elson D. [1971] The effect of erythromycin on peptide bond formation and the termination reaction FEBS Lett 15: 249-253.

Woods D.D. [1962] The biochemical mode of action of the sulphonamide drugs. J Gen Microbial 29: 687-702.

TOXOPLASMA GONDII : CHEMOTHERAPY

Hernan R. Chang* MB, MD, Dr Med
Department of Genetics and Microbiology
University of Geneva Medical School
9, avenue de Champel
1211 Geneva 4
Switzerland

Infection with *Toxoplasma gondii* is widespread and has been observed in man and in almost all warm-blooded animals. Most immunologically normal adults acutely infected with *T. gondii* present only self-limited symptoms and signs. This is in great contrast with the morbidity and mortality that is observed in children with congenital and acquired toxoplasmosis, and in immunocompromised patients, notably those affected by the acquired immune deficiency syndrome (AIDS). Prompt antimicrobial therapy is given to patients with the aim of inhibiting the replication of the parasite and to prevent or to reduce the tissue damage resulting from parasitic intracellular multiplication. This therapy, nevertheless, is inactive against the non-multiplying (extracellular) or metabolically inactive (cyst) form of the parasite. Therapy of toxoplasmosis is further complicated by the possibility of harmful effects of the drugs on the fetus during therapy of pregnant women infected for the first time with *T. gondii*. The high frequency of side effects observed in AIDS patients treated for toxoplasmic encephalitis may lead to withdrawal of therapy and this enhances the possibilities of recurrent disease. All these considerations, therefore, point out the need for safer alternatives in the therapy of toxoplasmosis.

During the past 50 years several active, clinically useful, antitoxoplasma compounds have been discovered by empirical screening. This practical approach was aided by the fact that most compounds previously used for Plasmodium were also found to be active against Toxoplasma. This approach, however, has often lead to a poor understanding of the exact mechanisms underlying the effects of the drugs against the parasite, the exception being, perhaps, the antifolates. Therefore, a more rational approach would be a preferable way to design more specific, improved, drugs in the future. Nonetheless, our knowledge on basic issues concerning the parasite, such as its mechanisms of invasion of host cells, metabolic pathways or the mechanisms and genes controlling tissue cyst formation, which could allow the

----

* Present address: Department of Microbiology, Faculty of Medicine, National University of Singapore, Lower Kent Ridge Road, Singapore 0511.

NATO ASI Series, Vol. H 78
Toxoplasmosis
Edited by Judith E. Smith
© Springer-Verlag Berlin Heidelberg 1993

identification of potential targets useful for chemotherapeutic intervention, is in its infancy.

Drugs active against the tachyzoite or endozoite form of the parasite must pass across the membranes of the host cell, the parasitophorous membrane, the parasitic plasmalemma and interfere with an essential process of the parasite. Drugs may also indirectly affect the parasites, e.g. by blocking a particular metabolic pathway in the host cells and, thereby, ceasing resources for normal intracellular development of the parasite. However, considering the eukaryotic nature of *T. gondii*, drugs which are toxic for the parasites are also potentially toxic for the host cells. There are some, already identified, parasitic metabolic pathways which are different in several aspects to those of the host cells and, therefore, potentially useful as targets for the development of a rational anti-parasitic therapy. The identification of further metabolic pathways, specially those unique to Toxoplasma, should be given top research priority in future studies.

Many *in vitro* and *in vivo* models of disease have been used in testing the activity of compounds against *T. gondii*. Standardization of the endpoints has not been achieved and this may vary according to the model used. One way to overcome these problems might be to install a repository center in which stabilates of reference strains would be kept and made available to the scientific community. Moreover, rules for standardization of the tests could be set up by a panel of experts.

DRUGS AFFECTING NUCLEIC ACID METABOLISM.- Scanty metabolism of nucleic acids is observed when *T. gondii* is extracellular. In contrast, during its intracellular growth and multiplication, a vigorous nucleic acid synthesis by the parasite takes place. A great number of 2,4-diaminopyrimidines, sulfa-derivatives, sulfones, and purine and pyrimidine analogues have some activity against *T. gondii*, suggesting the need for an untouched nucleic acid metabolism for parasitic growth. This heralds significant differences between the host's and parasite's metabolism which deserves further exploration.

ANTIFOLATES.- These drugs are currently divided into inhibitors of the dihydropteroate synthase (sulfonamides and sulfones) and inhibitors of the dihydrofolate reductase (2,4-diaminopyrimidines). The basis for the use of these drugs rests upon the fact that the metabolic machinery and enzymes of the parasite possess a higher affinity for the drugs than those of the host cells.

The synergistic combination of pyrimethamine, a dihiydrofolate reductase inhibitor, and sulfadiazine (or trisulfapyrimidines), a competitive inhibitor of the dihydropteroate synthase, is currently the most effective therapy for toxoplasmosis. This combination provides a sequential blockade of the folic acid metabolism and acts synergistically on *T. gondii* tachyzoites *in vitro* and *in vivo*, but not on the dormant cyst form of the parasite. Pyrimethamine-sulfadiazine and pyrimethamine-sulfadoxine has been used for the prevention and therapy of congenital toxoplasmosis both in pregnant women and after delivery with or without alternate treatment with spiramycin. Trimetrexate, an analogue of methotrexate, has been found to have an antitoxoplasmic effect *in vitro* and *in vivo* [Allegra *et al.*, 1987], but preliminary clinical studies have been disappointing. Piritrexim, another analogue of methotrexate, has limited activity on *T. gondii in vivo* but has been found to be synergistic with sulfadiazine both *in vitro* and in a murine model of acute toxoplasmosis [Kovacs *et al.*, 1988; Araujo *et al.*, 1987]. The antitoxoplasmic activity of dapsone (DDS, 4,4,'-diaminodiphenylsulfone), which is used in the treatment of Hansen's disease, has been recognised for more than 40 years [Summers, 1949]. In combination with pyrimethamine, however, the effect of DDS is less impressive than pyrimethamine-sulfadiazine in the treatment of animal toxoplasmosis. However, since DDS is better tolerated than sulfadiazine, its potential use for the prophylaxis or maintenance therapy of human toxoplasmic encephalitis deserves further study. Trimethoprim has poor activity on *T. gondii* but it synergizes with sulfamethoxazole. This combination (co-trimoxazole) has been found active in animal models of the disease by some authors but others have observed poor activity. Nevertheless, it has been used with success in the therapy of mild human toxoplasmosis.

PURINE METABOLISM.- *T. gondii* is unable to synthesize the purine ring de novo, which has been shown by the failure of radiolabeled glycine, formate and serine to label nucleic acid of the parasites in minimal defined medium. The purine bases hypoxanthine, guanine and adenine, the purine nucleosides inosine, adenosine, guanosine and xanthosine as well as ATP can be utilized by *T. gondii* as sources of purines. Of the purine salvage enzymes, adenosine kinase, adenine, guanine and adenosine deaminases, inosine and guanosine phosphorylases, and adenine, guanine, xanthine and hypoxanthine phosphoribosyltransferases have been reported for Toxoplasma [Krug *et al.*, 1989]. Adenosine arabinoside, a nucleoside analogue in which adenine is linked to arabinosine rather than ribose or deoxyribose, has been found to inhibit the growth of *T. gondii in vitro* at concentrations which had no toxic effect on the host cells [Pfefferkorn & Pfefferkorn, 1978].

PYRIMIDINE METABOLISM.- *T. gondii* is endowed with significant amounts of the enzyme uracil phosphoribosyltransferase, which catalyzes the conversion of uracil to uridylic acid, and therefore can incorporate radiolabeled uracil. The mammalian host cells do not contain this enzyme [Pfefferkorn & Pfefferkorn, 1977]. Fluoridine, 5-fluorodeoxyuridine and 5-fluorouracil, may act against *T. gondii* by the same pathway [Pfefferkorn, 1978]. 5-fluorouracil, following metabolism to deoxynucleotide 5-fluorodeoxyuridylate forms a stable covalent complex with thymidilate synthase, and N5N10 methylnetetrahydrofolate, the tetrahydrofolic acid coenzyme that catalyzes the reaction. This blockade is due to the high affinity to 5-fluorodeoxyuridylate for thymidilate synthethase. 5-fluorouracil and pyrimethamine act synergistically to inhibit the growth of *T. gondii in vitro* [Harris *et al.*, 1988]. Studies have shown that *T. gondii* is able to survive intracellularly without using uracil phosphoribosyltransferase, suggesting that the parasite does not require pyrimidine salvage to survive. The independence of *T. gondii* from pyrimidine salvage suggest that there is an adequately functioning pyrimidine synthesis machinery in the parasite.

Emimicyn, an antimicrobial product of a Streptomyces sp., which has been used as a veterinary anticoccidial, has potential antitoxoplasmic activity in infected human fibroblasts. Emimicyn is a good substrate as uracil for the uracil phosphoribosyltransferase of *T. gondii* and its incorporation into the nucleotide pool of *T. gondii* appears essential for its antitoxoplasma activity [Pfefferkorn *et al.*, 1989].

DRUGS INHIBITING PROTEIN SYNTHESIS.- Many antibiotics acting on bacterial ribosomes possess antitoxoplasma activity. Their mechanism of action on *T. gondii* is presently unknown but it may well be acting on the parasite mitochondrial ribosomes [H.R. Chang, unpublished results]. Some members of the families of macrolides, tetracyclines and clindamycin, have been found active on *T. gondii in vivo* and for some compounds also *in vitro* [Chang & Luft, 1986; Chang & Pechere, 1987; Chang & Pechere, 1988a; Chang *et al.*, 1988; Chang *et al.*, 1990a; Chang *et al.*, 1991; Araujo *et al.*, 1988; Araujo & Remington, 1974; Tabbara *et al.*, 1982]. Tetracycline, chlortetracycline and dimethylchlortetracycline have been assessed for their activity in acute murine toxoplasmosis, but the results of these studies yielded disparate results. It appears that with the exception of the semi-synthetic analogue minocycline [Chang *et al.*, 1991], none of the ribosome-binding antibiotics possess a very potent antitoxoplasmic activity.

VETERINARY ANTICOCCIDIALS.- In addition to emimycin, several veterinary anticoccidials were active *in vitro* against *T. gondii* but they were inactive against the parasite in the mouse model or extremely toxic for the animals [H.R. Chang, unpublished results]. Arprinocid, a veterinary anticoccidial agent, and its main metabolite arprinocid-1-N-oxide have been found to exert a cidal effect on *T. gondii in vitro* and in murine toxoplasmosis [Luft, 1986; Pfefferkorn *et al.* 1988]. *In vivo*, arprinocid is converted into arprinocid-1-N-oxide which seems to be the therapeutically active form. Their mechanism of action on *T. gondii* are unknown. Arprinocid-1-N-oxide has been found active on metabolically active cysts of *T. gondii in vitro* [Huskinson-Mark *et al.*, 1991].

1,2,4-TRIOXANES AND QINGHAOSU.- Some derivatives of qinghaosu, a natural product obtained from Artemisia annua, a plant which originates from China, and used in the therapy of severe malaria, were previously found inactive against *T. gondii* in the animal model and poorly active *in vitro* [Chang & Pechere, 1988b] . However, other studies suggest that these compounds have an activity on the parasite *in vitro* [Ou-Yang *et al.*, 1990]. All these products are characterized by the presence of a 1,2,4-trioxane ring in their structure. It has been found that synthetic 1,2,4-trioxanes are also active against *T. gondii in vitro* [Chang *et al.*, 1989]. Further work with these compounds are required to unravel their mechanism of action and assess their potential usefulness in the therapy of *T. gondii* infections.

HYDROXYNAPHTOQUINONES.- Hydroxynaphtoquinones, compounds known for many years as antimalarials, are also active against *T. gondii*. A newly synthesized member of this familiy of compounds, 566C80, has been recently reported to be active against *T. gondii in vitro* and *in vivo* [Araujo *et al.*, 1991]. Further studies claim a parasiticidal effect of this compound on metabolically active *T. gondii* cysts (metabolically inactive cysts are not affected), *in vitro* and *in vivo* [Araujo *et al.*, 1992]. The mechanism of action of this hydroxynaphtoquinone on *T. gondii* is unknown.

CYTOKINES. IFN-γ alone or in combination with several drugs has been found to protect mice in models of Toxoplasma infection [McCabe *et al.*, 1984; Israelski & Remington, 1991]. Interleukin-1 and tumor necrosis factor (TNF), have been found either alone or in combination to significantly protect mice against a lethal challenge of *T. gondii* [Chang *et al.*, 1990b]. Recently, the presence of significant amounts of mRNA for TNF in the brains of C57B6L/J (H-2b) mice with chronic toxoplasmic encephalitis has been demonstrated. Uninfected mice did not present TNF mRNA transcripts [Chang *et al.*, 1992]. In situ hybridization, showed that the mRNA was associated with perivascular inflammatory leukocytes, however TNF protein, as detected by immunohistochemistry was localized on the surface of the ependymal cells and in the tissue *T. gondii* cysts [Chang *et al.*, 1992]. It is difficult to comprehend the reason for this, but its presence suggests a role for TNF in the development of the cysts and in their control. Further evidence for this role was provided by the observation that the number of *T. gondii* cysts increased when mice received an infusion of anti-TNF antibodies whereas administration of recombinant TNF reduced the number of parasitic cysts in the brains of mice. Another group of researchers has obtained data indicating that polymorphisms in the TNF gene in mice correlate with resistance to toxoplasmic encephalitis and with the levels of TNF mRNA in the infected brain tissue [Freund *et al.*, 1992]. At this time it has not been established whether or not modulation of cytokine production would play a major role in the therapy of *T. gondii* infection.

Allegra CJ, Kovacs JA, Drake JC, Swan JC Chabner BA, Masur H (1987) Potent *in vitro* and *in vivo* antitoxoplasma activity of the lipid-soluble antifolate trimetrexate. J Clin Invest 79:478-482.

Araujo FG, Remington JS, (1974) Effect of clindamycin on acute and chronic toxoplasmosis in mice. Antimicrob Agents Chemother 5:647-651.

Araujo FG, Guptill DR, Remington JS (1987) In vivo activity of piritrexim against *Toxoplasma gondii*. J Inf Dis 156:828-830.

Araujo FG, Guptill DR, Remington JS (1988) Azithromycin, a macrolide with potent activity against *Toxoplasma gondii*. Antimicrob Agents Chemother 32:755-757.

Araujo FG, Huskinson J, Remington JS (1991) Remarkable *in vitro* and *in vivo* activities of the hydroxynaphtoquinone 566C80 against tachyzoites and tissue cysts of *Toxoplasma gondii*. Antimicrob Agents Chemother 35:293-299.

Araujo FG, Huskinson-Mark J, Gutteridge WE, Remington JS (1992) *In vitro* and *in vivo* activities of the hydroxynapthoquinone 566C80 against the cyst form of *Toxoplasma gondii*. Antimicrob Agents Chemother 36:326-330.

Chan J, Luft BJ (1986) Activity of roxithromycin (RU 28965), a macrolide, against *Toxoplasma gondii* infection in mice. Antimicrob Agents Chemother 30:323-324.

Chang HR, Pechere JCF (1987) Effect of roxithromycin on acute toxoplasmosis in mice. 31:1147-1149.

Chang HR, Pechere JC (1988a) *In vitro* effects of four macrolides (roxithromycin, spiramycin, azithromycin [CP-62,993], and A-56268) on *Toxoplasma gondii*. Antimicrob Agents Chemother 32:524-529.

Chang HR, Pechere JC (1988b) Arteether, a qinghaosu derivative in toxoplasmosis. Trans Roy Soc Trop Med Hyg 82:867.

Chang HR, Rudareanu FC, Pechere JC (1988) Activity of A-56268 (TE-031), a new macrolide against *Toxoplasma gondii* in mice. J Antimicrob Agents Chemother 22:359-361.

Chang HR, Jefford CW, Pechere JC (1989) *In vitro* effects of three new 1,2,4-trioxanes (pentatroxane, thiahexatroxane, and hexatroxanone) on

Toxoplasma gondii. Antimicrob Agents Chemother 33:1748-1752.

Chang HR, Comte R, Pechere JC (1990) *In vitro* and *in vivo* effects of doxycycline on *Toxoplasma gondii.* Antimicrob Agents Chemother 34:775-780.

Chang HR, Grau GE, Pechere JC (1990) Role of TNF and IL-1 infections with *Toxoplasma gondii.* Immunology 69:33-37.

Chang HR, Comte R, Piguet PF, Pechere JC (1991) Activity of minocycline against *Toxoplasma gondii* in mice. J Antimicrob Chemother 27:639-645.

Chang HR, Pechere JC, Piguet PF (1992) Role of tumour necrosis factor in murine chronic toxoplasmic *Toxoplasma gondii* encephalitis. Immunol Infect Dis 2:61-68.

Freund YR, Slargato G, Jacob CO, Suzuki Y, Remington JS (1992) Polymorphisms in tumor necrosis factor α (TNF-α) gene correlate with murine resistance to development of toxoplasmic encephalitis and with levels of TNF-α mRNA in infected brain tissue. J Exp Med 175:683-688.

Harris C, Salgo MP, Tanowitz HB, Wittner M (1988) *In vitro* assessment of antimicrobial agents against Toxoplasma gondii. J Infect Dis 157:14-22.

Huskinson-Mark J, Araujo FG, Remington JS (1991) Evaluation of the effect of drugs on the cyst form of *Toxoplasma gondii.* J Infect Dis 164:170-177.

Israelski D, Remington JS (1991) Activity of γ interferon in combination with pyrimethamine or clindamycin in the treatment of murine toxoplasmosis. Eur J Clin Microbiol Infect Dis 9:358-360.

Kovacs JA, Allegra CJ, Swan JC, Drake J, Parrillo JE, Chabner BA, Masur H (1988) Potent antipneumocystis and antitoxoplasma activities of piritrexim, a lipid-soluble antifolate. Antimicrob Agents Chemother 32:430-433.

Krug EC, Marr JJ, Berens RL (1989) Purine metabolism in *Toxoplasma gondii.* J Biol Chem 264:10601-10807.

Luft BJ (1986) Potent in vivo activity of arprinocid, a purine analogue, against murine toxoplasmosis. J Infect Dis 154:692-694.

McCabe RE, Luft BJ, Remington JS (1984) Effect of murine interferon γ in toxoplasmosis. J Infect Dis 150:961-962.

Ou-Yang K, Krug EC, Marr JJ, Berens RL (1990) Inhibition of growth of *Toxoplasma gondii* by qinghaosu and derivatives. Antimicrob Agents Chemother 34:1961-1965.

Pfefferkorn ER (1978) *Toxoplasma gondii*: the enzymic defect of a mutant resistant to 5-fluorodeoxyuridine. Exp Parasitol 44:26-35.

Pfefferkorn ER, Pfefferkorn LC (1977) Specific labeling of intracellular *Toxoplasma gondii* with uracil. J Protozool 24:449-453.

Pfefferkorn ER, Pfefferkorn LC (1978) The biochemical basis for resistance to adenine arabinoside in a mutant of *T. gondii.* J Parasitol 64:488-492.

Pfefferkorn ER, Eckel ME, McAdams E (1988) *Toxoplasma gondii*: *in vitro* and *in vivo* studies with a mutant resistant to arprinocid-N-oxide. Exp Parasitol 65:282-289.

Pfefferkorn ER, Eckel ME, McAdams E (1989) *Toxoplasma gondii*: the biochemical basis of resistance to emimycin. Exp Parasitol 69:129-139.

Summers WA (1949) The effects of oral administration of aureomycin, sulfathiazole, sulfamerazine, and 4,4-diaminodiphenylsulfone on toxoplasmosis in mice. Amer J Trop Med 29:889-893.

Tabbara KF, Sakuragi S, O'Connor GR (1982) Minocycline in the chemotherapy of murine toxoplasmosis. Parasitology 84:297-302.

DIAGNOSIS OF *TOXOPLASMA GONDII* INFECTIONS BY MOLECULAR DETECTION

E. Schoondermark-van de Ven, J. Galama, W. Camps
J. Meuwissen, W. Melchers
University Hospital Nijmegen
Department of Medical Microbiology
P.O. Box 9101
6500 HB Njmegen
The Netherlands

Abstract

In this report the applicability of *in situ* hybridization (ISH) and the polymerase chain reaction (PCR) is described for the diagnosis of toxoplasmosis.

The presence of *T. gondii* cysts in the brain of experimentally infected mice was clearly demonstrated by ISH using digoxigenin labeled oligonucleotide probes directed against the B1 gene. With this technique, the parasite could be localized within the morphological structure of the infected tissue.

A novel PCR assay was developed with the small subunit ribosomal RNA (16S-like rRNA) as a target. The abundance of rRNA target sequences enabled a single parasite to be detected with this RNA based amplification system.

The usefulness of these molecular assays for the diagnosis of *T. gondii* infections will be further outlined in this report.

Introduction

Diagnosis of toxoplasmosis is problematic both in congenital infection and in recurrent infection, as occurs in immunocompromised patients. Serology is frequently unreliable, and more direct approaches to detect *T. gondii* in clinical specimens by microscopy, antigen detection, or inoculation of samples into mice or tissue culture are either insensitive or time-consuming [Remington & Desmonts, 1990]. Since early treatment is mandatory in such infections, we, and other research groups, have sought to develop alternative diagnosis by molecular techniques.

NATO ASI Series, Vol. H 78
Toxoplasmosis
Edited by Judith E. Smith
© Springer-Verlag Berlin Heidelberg 1993

In situ hybridization (ISH) has become an established technique for the detection and identification of infectious agents in diagnostic microbiology and pathology (Warford & Lauder, 1991). The method preserves morphological structures and permits the exact localization of *T. gondii* within the tissue. The ISH differs from other molecular techniques in that the nucleic acids are not isolated from the clinical sample. In contrast to many other microorganisms, conventional molecular hybridization methods as dot-spot and Southern-blot analysis have rarely been applied to the detection of *T. gondii*. This is, most probably, due to the low sensitivity of these assays. In fact, Weiss et al. (1991) described a detection level of 10,000 parasites using Southern-blot analysis, too high to be useful in diagnosis of toxoplasmosis. Over the last few years much attention focused on the use of PCR for the detection of *T. gondii*. Although theoretically a single parasite can be detected, in practice, the detection level is about 10 parasites (Burg et al., 1989; Weiss et al., 1991). Thus, even in some instances of proven infection, detection of *T. gondii* in cerebrospinal or amniotic fluid may fail due to low densities of parasites (Cristina et al., 1992; Schoondermark-Van de Ven et al., 1992c). Therefore the sensitivity of the PCR should be increased. Computer alignment studies of ribosomal RNA (rRNA) sequences have revealed the existence of regions with highly conserved sequences among eukaryotes but also regions which display sequence variability (Gray et al., 1984). This should allow the selection of *T. gondii* specific primers for the PCR. Besides the unique sequence features, rRNA molecules are present in all ribosomes. Thus rRNA is naturally present in high copy number, up to 10,000 molecules per parasite (Waters & McCutchan, 1990), and provides a target for a highly sensitive PCR assay. We have therefore recently elucidated the sequence of the complete 16S-like rRNA of *T. gondii* (Schoondermark-Van de Ven et al., 1992b). We selected *T. gondii* specific primers and examined the specificity and sensitivity of this primer set for the detection of *T. gondii*.

Materials and methods
In situ hybridization
The ISH assay was tested on brain of mice infected with the cyst forming *T. gondii* strain T626. The mouse brains were harvested 3 months after infection, fixed in buffered formalin, embedded in paraffin and processed for ISH as previously described (Melchers et al., 1989). The deparaffinized sections were treated with proteinase K for 10 minutes to obtain an optimal equilibrium between probe accessibility to the cell and tissue deterioration.

Hybridization was performed with an oligonucleotide probe (5'-GGCGACCAATCTGCGAATACACC-3') directed against the B1 gene (position 831-853, Burg et al., 1989). The probe was tailed with digoxigenin-dUTP (Boehringer-Mannheim) with terminal deoxynucleotidyl transferase (TdT) according to standard conditions (Ausubel et al., 1989), and diluted in the hybridization mixture (Melchers et al., 1989) at a concentration of 3 ng/ul. Hybridization, washing and immunological detection was performed according to the manufacturer instructions, modified for ISH (Boehringer-Mannheim).

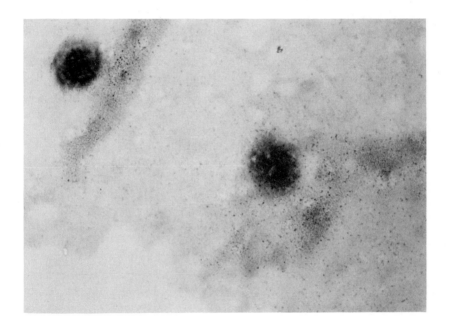

Figure 1. Demonstration of *T. gondii* bradyzoites in infected mouse brain by *in situ* hybridization using a digoxigenin tailed oligonucleotide directed against the B1-gene.

Polymerase chain reaction

The complete nucleotide sequence of the small subunit ribosomal RNA of *T. gondii* was elucidated (EMBL Acc.nr X65508, Schoondermark-Van de Ven et al., 1992b). *T. gondii* specific primers were selected using the

CAOS/CAMMSA computer analysis program. One primer was selected in the second variable region (V2: 5'-GTTGACTTCGGTCTGCGACG-3') and the other primer in the third variable region (V3: 5'-TTCCAATCACTAGAAATGAA-3') of the 16S-like rRNA of *T. gondii*.

cDNA synthesis with the V3 primer was performed as previously described (Zoll et al., 1992). The thermal profile involved 40 cycles of denaturation at 94^0 for 1 min, primer annealing at 42^0 for 30 sec, and primer extension at 72^0 for 2 min, and resulted in the amplification of a 238 bp product. The amplified products were analysed by agarose gel electrophoresis and Southern-blot analysis as previously described (Van de Ven et al., 1991).

T. gondii parasites were grown on HEp-2 cells and RNA was isolated by the RNAzolB method (Cinna/Biotecx, Veenendaal, The Netherlands).

Results

1. *In situ* hybridization

As shown in Figure 1, ISH on brains infected with *T. gondii* resulted in the hybridization with the cysts. A clear purple granular hybridization signal can be observed specifically in the bradyzoites. No substantional back-ground staining or staining of the cyst wall was observed, demonstrating the specificity of the probe and the <DIG> detection system.

2. Polymerase chain reaction

a. Sensitivity of the PCR assay

Both chromosomal DNA and undegraded rRNA were isolated from purified T. gondii parasites (Figure 2). This enables a direct comparison in sensitivit between the amplification of rDNA and reverse transcribed rRNA. To determine the sensitivity of the PCR assay, serial dilutions of purified *T. gondii* nucleic acids were made. Without prior transcribing the RNA, a sensitivity of 10 pg was obtained, as detected by gel electrophoresis and ethidium bromide staining (Figure 3). This corresponds to approximately 100 parasites. However, when the rRNA was first transcribed by reverse transcriptase into cDNA, the detection level was 0.1 pg, corresponding to a single parasite (Figure 3). Using a rRNA based PCR assay it is thus possible to detect the nucleic acid content, equivalent to a single *T. gondii* parasite by agarose gel electrophoresis. In fact the sensitivity is approximately a factor 10 higher when Southern-blot analysis is performed (data not shown).

b. Specificity of the PCR assay

The specificity of the V2/V3 primer combination was investigated with 5 characterized *T. gondii* strains (RH and T626 from Nijmegen, The Netherlands and, C, P, and RH, kindly provided by dr. J. Boothroyd, Stanford, USA), and 12 wild-type isolates from European patients. From all strains a specific fragment of 238 bp was generated with the V2/V3 primer set (data not shown).

No specific amplification was observed when the primer set was tested with human DNA nor with a broad spectrum of microorganisms (N=32) among which microorganisms causing congenital, cerebral, and opportunistic infections and parasites related to *T. gondii*.

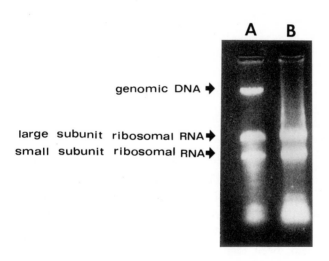

Figure 2. Isolation of total nucleic acids (A) or RNA (B) of *T. gondii*.

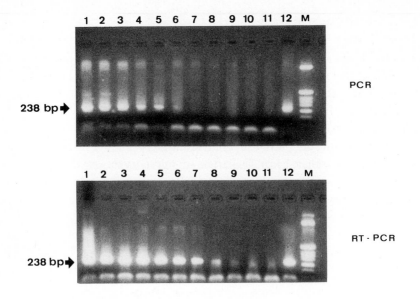

Figure 3. Amplification of *T. gondii* rDNA directly (top) or after reverse transcription of the rRNA into cDNA (bottom) in a sample containing total nucleic acids.
Lanes 1-10: 100 ng, 10 ng, 1 ng, 100 pg, 10 pg, 1 pg, 100 fg, 10 fg, 1 fg, and 0.1 fg of *T. gondii* DNA. Lane 11: negative control (distilled water), and lane 12: 30 ng *T. gondii* DNA (positive control).

Discussion

PCR has already proven its usefulness for the detection of *T. gondii* in brain biopsy samples and cerebrospinal fluid of immunocompromised patients with cerebral toxoplasmosis (Holliman et al., 1991; Lebech et al., 1992; Van de Ven et al., 1991; Schoondermark-Van de Ven et al., 1992a). Congenital toxoplasmosis has also been demonstrated by PCR in amniotic fluid, cerebrospinal fluid, and post-mortem material (Grover et al., 1990; Van de Ven et al., 1991; Schoondermark-Van de Ven et al., 1992c; Verhofstede et al., 1990). Besides this, PCR can be applied to both fresh and formalin fixed clinical material which makes transportation and storage of materials much easier (Van de Ven et al., 1991).

Although these PCR assays could detect as few as ten parasites, in some instances PCR failed to detect *T. gondii* in toxoplasma infections as proven by parasite isolation (Cristina et al., 1992). This negative PCR result might be caused by the presence of components in the clinical sample which inhibit the enzymatic amplification. However, the possibility that the detection limit of 10 parasites, as obtained by PCR, is not sensitive enough to detect a *T. gondii* infection cannot be excluded. In fact, the latter possibility is supported by our experience in a monkey model of congenital toxoplasmosis: using the PCR on the BI gene, *T. gondii* could not be detected in amniotic fluid samples which were positive by mouse inoculation. These samples, however, were positive by a nested PCR assay (Schoondermark-Van de Ven et al., 1992c). The rRNA based amplification may be an approach to improve the sensitivity of PCR. By making use of the abundance of rRNA target sequences, a sensitivity can be achieved that is comparable to that of nested PCR. And indeed, prelimenary results show that the rRNA-PCR is as sensitive as nested PCR for the detection of *T. gondii* in clinical specimens. For diagnostic applications, a single (rRNA-PCR) has the preference since care must be exercised to avoid contamination. The applicability of this rRNA-PCR on clinical specimens is currently investigated.

The necessity of ISH for the detection of *T. gondii* may not be that obvious, but in specific cases the test can be a valuable diagnostic tool. The diagnosis of cerebral toxoplasmosis is complicated. The results on the detection of *T. gondii* in cerebrospinal fluid of AIDS patients by PCR are very promising (Schoondermark-Van de Ven et al., 1992a), but still, in some patients a brain biopsy is inevitably required for diagnosis. Discrimination between latent (cyst stage) and active (tachyzoite stage) cerebral toxoplasmosis in a brain biopsy is only possible by microscopical examination. Identification may be assisted by the use of immunofluorescence, a technique which is as specific and sensitive as ISH but much faster and less laborious. The value of ISH is therefore not directly as a diagnostic tool for toxoplasmosis but rather in basic research, for instance, in the study of specific gene-expression in the bradyzoite and tachyzoite stages of infection and the metabolic differences during the parasite life cycle.

Acknowledgement

This research was supported by grant 28-1604 of the Prevention Fund, The Netherlands.

References

Ausubel FM, Brent R, Kingston RE, Moore DD, Seidman JG, Smith JA, Struhl K (1989) Current protocols in molecular biology. John Wiley & Sons, Inc., New York.

Burg JL, Grover CM, Pouletty P, Boothroyd JC (1989) Direct and sensitive detection of a pathogenic protozoan, *Toxoplasma gondii*, by polymerase chain reaction. J Clin Microbiol 27:1787-1792.

Cristina N, Derouin F, Pelloux H, Pierce R, Cesbron-Delauw MF, Abroise-Thomas P (1992) Polymerase chain reaction detection of *Toxoplasma gondii* in AIDS patients using the repetative sequence TGR1$_e$. Path Biol 40:52-55.

Holliman RE, Johnson JD, Gillespie SH, Johnson MA, Squire SB, Savva D (1991) New methods in the diagnosis and management of cerebrospinal toxoplasmosis associated with the aquired immune deficiency syndrome. J Infect 22:281-285.

Gray MW, Sankoff D, Cerdergren RJ (1984) On the evolutionary descent of microorganisms and organelles: A global phylogeny based on highly conserved structural core in small subunit ribosomal RNA. Nucleic Acid Res 12:5837-5852.

Grover CM, Thulliez P, Remington JS, Boothroyd JC (1990) Rapid prenatal diagnosis of congenital *Toxoplasma* infection by using polymerase chain reaction and amniotic fluid. J Clin Microbiol 28:2297-2301.

Lebech M, Lebech A, Nelsing S, Vuust J, Mathiesen L, Petersen E (1992) Detection of *Toxoplasma gondii* DNA by polymerase chain reaction in cerebrospinal fluid from AIDS patients with cerebral toxoplasmosis. J Infect Dis 165:982-983.

Melchers WJG, Herbrink P, Quint WGV (1989) DNA detection techniques for routine diagnosis of infections. In Bullock G, Leathem A, Velzen van D (eds.): "Techniques in diagnostic pathology." Academic Press Limited, London 1:151-171.

Remington JS, Desmonts(1990) Toxoplasmosis. In Remington JS, Klein JO (eds.): "Infectious diseases of the fetus and the newborn infant." W.B. Saunders Company, Philadelphia, pp:89-195.

Schoondermark-van de Ven E, Galama J, Kraaijeveld C, van Druten J, Meuwissen J, Melchers W (1992a) Diagnostic value of the polymerase chain reaction of *T. gondii* in cerebrospinal fluid of patients with AIDS. Clin Infect Dis (in press).

Schoondermark-van de Ven E, Galama J, Melchers W (1992b) Sequence of the small subunit rRNA gene of *Toxoplasma gondii* and its use in phylogenetic analysis Submitted for publication.

Schoondermark-van de Ven E, Melchers W, Galama J, Camps W, Eskes T, Meuwissen (1992c) Congenital toxoplasmosis: An experimental study in Rhesus monkeys for transmission and prenatal diagnosis. Submitted for publication.

Ven van de E, Melchers W, Galama J, Camps W, Meuwissen J (1991) Identification of *Toxoplasma gondii* by B1 gene amplification. J Clin Microbiol 29:2120-2124.

Verhofstede C, Renterheim L, Plum J, Vanderscheuren S, Verhaesbrouck P (1990) Congenital toxoplasmosis and TORCH. Lancet 336:622-623.

Waters AP, McCutchan TF (1990) Ribosomal RNA: Nature's own polymerase-amplified target for diagnosis. Parasitol Today 6:56-59.

Warford A, Lauder I (1991) In situ hybridization in perspective. J Clin Pathol 44:177-181.

Weiss LM, Udem SA, Salgo M, Tanowitz HB, Wittner M (1991) Sensitive and specific detection of *Toxoplasma* DNA in an experimental murine model: Use of *Toxoplasma gondii*-specific cDNA and the polymerase chain reaction. J Infect Dis 163:180-186.

Zoll GJ, Melchers WJG, Kopecka H, Jambroes G, Poel van der HJA, Galama JMD (1992) General primer-mediated polymerase chain reaction for detection of enteroviruses: Application for diagnostic routine and persistent infections. J Clin Microbiol 30:160-165.

USE OF *TOXOPLASMA GONDII* RECOMBINANT ANTIGENS FOR DIAGNOSIS AND SEROEPIDEMIOLOGY

A.M. Tenter and A.M. Johnson[1]
Institut fur Parasitologie
Tierarztliche Hockschule Hannover
Bunteweg 17
3000 Hannover 71
Germany

Introduction

The production of antigens for serological tests used in the diagnosis of infections with *T. gondii* has been complicated by the fact that the *T. gondii* life cycle stages from which these antigens are derived are obligately intracellular. Therefore, traditional antigen preparations, which are usually derived from parasites grown in tissue cultures or the peritoneal cavities of mice, are inevitably contaminated with at least some host material. In addition, such antigen preparations are expensive and lack standardization.

In an attempt to overcome these problems, we have cloned, sequenced and characterized fragments of two single-copy genes, termed *H4* and *H11*, that encode antigenic polypeptides of *T. gondii* [Johnson and Illana, 1991]. The messenger RNAs of the *H4* and *H11* genes consist of about 1300 and 1900 nt, respectively, and occur in low abundances in the endozoite stage of *T. gondii*. The native endozoite polypeptides encoded by the *H4* and *H11* genes have apparent molecular weights of 25000 and 41000, respectively. To examine the diagnostic potential of the recombinant H4 and H11 polypeptides the *H4* and *H11* gene fragments were subcloned from a Lambda gt11 expression library into the plasmid pGEX-1N. The recombinant polypeptides were then expressed as glutathione-*S*-transferase fusion polypeptides [Tenter and Johnson, 1991] and used to develop Enzyme-linked Immunosorbent Assays

---

[1]Department of Microbiology, University of Technology, Sydney, Westbourne Street, Gore Hill, New South Wales 2065, Australia

NATO ASI Series, Vol. H 78
Toxoplasmosis
Edited by Judith E. Smith
© Springer-Verlag Berlin Heidelberg 1993

(ELISAs) for diagnosis of *T. gondii* infections in intermediate and definitive host.

A study on recombinant polypeptides for the diagnosis of malaria showed that an ELISA using a mixture of three recombinant polypeptides of *Plasmodium falciparum* is more sensitive than ELISAs using single *P. falciparum* polypeptides [Srivastava et al. 1989]. Therefore, we evaluated the quality of ELISAs using either *H4* or *H11* only and of an ELISA using a mixture of *H4* and *H11* with respect to their usefulness for the diagnosis of *T. gondii* infections and for seroepidemiological surveys [Tenter and Johnson, 1991; Johnson et al. 1992; Tenter et al. 1992]. These recombinant *T. gondii* ELISAs were then compared with a laboratory produced ELISA using a traditional antigen preparation derived from *T. gondii* endozoites for detection of *T. gondii* specific antibodies in humans, sheep and cats [Tenter and Johnson, 1991; Tenter et al., 1992]. In addition, the recombinant *T. gondii* ELISAs were compared with a range of commerical ELISAs for the diagnosis of acute toxoplasmosis in humans [Johnson et al. 1992] and with an indirect fluorescent antibody test (IFAT), a direct agglutination test (DA), and the Sabin-Feldman dye test (DT), for the screening of large numbers of cat sera in epidemiological surveys. These results are reviewed here.

Results and Discussion

Table 1 lists the definitions and determinations of test characteristics calculated for the comparisons described above [Griner et al. 1981; Köbberrling et al. 1984].

Sensitivity and specificity

The operating characteristics determined in most studies evaluating serological tests are sensitivity and specificity. These two characteristics are required to determine the accuracy of the test under study and to decide whether or not it is useful to select this test for diagnosis or screening [Griner et al. 1981]. The knowledge of the sensitivity of a test provides information on the likelihood that the test result will be positive when the human or animal tested is infected

TABLE 1. Definitions and calculations of characteristics of diagnostic tests

Test characteristic	Definition	Formula
Sensitivity*	the probability that the test will be positive when the infection is present	true positives/ (true positives + false negatives)
Specificity*	the probability that the test will be negative when the infection is present	true negatives/ (true negatives + false positives)
Positive predictive factor**	the diagnostic value of the test with respect to its predictive accuracy for detecting the infection	sensitivity/ (sensitivity + 1 - specificity)
Negative predictive factor**	the diagnostic value of the test with respect to its predictive accuracy for excluding the infection	specificity/ (specificity + 1 - sensitivity
Positive predictive value*	the probability that the infection is present when the test is positive	true positives/ (true positives + false positives
Negative predictive value*	the probability that the infection is not present when the test is negative	true negatives/ (true negatives + false negatives)

*   Griner et al. [1991]
**   Kobberling et al. [1984]

with *T. gondii* while the knowledge of the specificity of a test provides information on the likelihood that the test result will be negative when the human or animal is not infected with *T. gondii*. In our studies the recombinant *T. gondii* ELISAs proved to be highly specific for anti-*T. gondii* antibodies [Tenter and Johnson, 1991; Johnson et al. 1992; Tenter et al. 1992] and consistent with the results of Srivastava et al. [1989], the ELISA using a mixture of *H4* and *H11* had a higher sensitivity than those using single *H4* and *H11* (Table 2).

TABLE 2. Comparison of ELISAs using recombinant antigens with an ELISA using antigens derived from *T. gondii* endozoites

Statistics	H4	H11	H4 and H11	Endozoites
Sheep				
Sensitivity (%)	79	43	79	100
Specificity (%)	100	100	100	100
Predictive factor				
- positive	1.00	1.00	1.00	1.00
- negative	0.83	0.64	0.83	1.00
Predictive value (%)				
- positive	100	100	100	100
- negative	80	60	80	100
(54% prevalence)				
Humans				
Sensitivity (%)	54	61	81	97
Specificity (%)	100	100	100	100
Predictive factor				
- positive	1.00	1.00	1.00	1.00
- negative	0.68	0.72	0.84	0.97
Predictive value (%)				
- positive	-	-	100	100
- negative	-	-	88	98
(43% prevalence)				
Cats				
Sensitivity (%)	85	62	94	95
Specificity (%)	99	98	99	100
Predictive factor				
- positive	0.99	0.97	0.99	1.00
- negative	0.87	0.72	0.94	0.95
Predictive value (%)				
- positive	98	97	98	100
- negative	93	71	94	95
(48% prevalence)				

Predictive values

As shown in Table 1 sensitivity is calculated from the group of infected humans or animals while specificity is calculated from the group of non-infected humans or animals. However, when epidemiological surveys are to be carried out it is usually not known which of the humans or animals are truly infected and which are truly non-infected. Thus, in these situations the major questions are: What is the likelihood that an infection with *T. gondii* is present when the test result is positive and what is the likelihood that an infection with *T. gondii* is absent when the test result is negative? To answer these questions it is important to know the positive and negative predictive values of the test [Griner et al., 1981; Köbberling, 1982]. Unlike sensitivity and specificity, which are constant operating characteristics as long as the test conditions are not altered, predictive values depend on the pre-test probability of infection in the group of humans or animals tested [Griner et al. 1981; Köbberling, 1982; Köbberling et al. 1984]. In our analysis, we calculated predictive values for prevalences of *T. gondii* infection in human, sheep and cat populations varying between 43 and 54% (Table 2).

TABLE 3. Comparison of the recombinant H4/H11 ELISA with different tests using antigen preparations of *T. gondii* endozoites for diagnosis of *T. gondii* infections in cats

	H4 and H11	Endozoites			
		ELISA	DT	DA	IFAT
Sensitivity (%)	84	100	95	100	95
Specificity (%)	100	100	95	89	78
Predictive factor					
- positive	1.00	1.00	0.95	0.90	0.81
- negative	1.00	0.97	0.95	1.00	0.94

$PPV = p\,c\,/\,[p\,c + (1 - p)\,(1 - c)]$
$NPV = (1 - p)\,c'\,/\,[(1 - p)\,c' + p\,(1 - c')]$.

Predictive factors

We are about to commence a large-scale seroepidemiological study on *T. gondii* infections in cats and sheep in Northern Germany, but have little information on the prevalence of *T. gondii* infection in Northern Germany at present. Therefore, we also calculated the positive and negative predictive factors of the tests compared here (Tables 2 and 3). These test characteristics are independent of the prevalence and describe the diagnostic value of a test with respect to the profit of predictive accuracy gained by the test result [Köbberling et al., 1984]. The recombinant *T. gondii* ELISA using the mixture of H4 and H11 showed high positive and negative predictive factors of ≥ 0.99 and ≥ 0.83, respectively. Hence this ELISA appears to be a very suitable diagnostic method both for detecting and for excluding infections with *T. gondii*. When the positive predictive factor (c) and negative predictive factor (c') are known it is possible to calculate positive predictive values (PPV) and negative predictive values (NPV) for any prevalence (p) of infection using the following formulae of Köbberling et al. [1984]:

Hence, the knowledge of the predictive factors of the recombinant *T. gondii* ELISA will now enable us to calculate its predictive values for any prevalence of *T. gondii* infection in human, sheep and cat populations and will thereby provide valuable information on the interpretation of results obtained by this test in epidemiological surveys.

Acknowledgements

This study was supported in part by a grant from Lower Saxony (Forschungsmittel des Landes Niedersachsen). The production and use of the recombinant antigens described here are covered by a patent (PK 1679).

References

Griner, P.F., Mayewski, R.J., Mushlin, A.I., Greenland, P. [1981] Selection and interpretation of diagnostic tests and procedures. Ann Int Med 94: 553-600.

Johnson, A.M., Illana, S. [1991] Cloning of *Toxoplasma gondii* gene fragments encoding diagnostic antigens. Gene 99: 127-132.

Johnson, A.M., Roberts, H., Tenter, A.M. [1992] Evaluation of a recombinant antigen ELISA for the diagnosis of acute toxoplamosis and comparison with traditional antigen ELISAs. J Med Microbiol: in press.

Köbberling, J. [1982] Der prädiktive Wert diagnostischer Maßnahman. Dtsch Med Wschr 107 591-595.

Köbberling, J., Richter, K., Tillil, H. [1984] The predictive factor - a method to simplify Bayes' formula and its application to diagnostic procedures. Klin Wschr 62: 586-592.

Srivastava, I.K., Takacs, B., Casper, P., Certa, V., McGregor, I.A., Scaife, J., Perrin, L.H. [1989] Recombinant polypeptides for serology of malaria. Trans R Soc Trop Med Hyg 83: 317-321.

Tenter, A.M., Johnson, A.M., [1991] Recognition of recombinant *Toxoplasma gondii* antigens by human sera in an ELISA. Parasitol. Res. 77: 197-203.

Tenter, A.M., Vietmeyer, C., Johnson, A.M. [1992] Development of ELISAs based on recombinant antigens for the detection of *Toxoplasma gondii* specific antibodies in sheep and cats. Vet Parasitol: in press.

PROGRESS TOWARDS THE DEVELOPMENT OF A VACCINE AGAINST CONGENITAL TOXPLAMOSIS: IDENTIFICATION OF PROTECTIVE ANTIGENS AND THE SELECTION OF APPROPRIATE ADJUVANTS

J. Alexander, C.W. Roberts & J.M. Brewer
Department of Immunology
University of Strathclyde
The Todd Centre
31 Taylor Street
GLASGOW G4 0NR

Summary

We have recently established that vertical disease transmission from the mother to the foetus, as in humans and sheep, only occurs in BALB/c mice infected with *Toxoplasma gondii* for first time during pregnancy. Thus a previous infection generally gives life long immunity, as ideally, would an effective vaccine. Of three major fractions harvested from RH strain tachyzoites (membrane, soluble and excretory/secretory) the soluble fraction was found the most effective in reducing mortality and cyst burdens in adult mice. Further studies indicated that the choice of adjuvant could enhance this effect. Entrapment within non-ionic surfactant vesicles (NISV), but not Freund's Complete Adjuvant, significantly enhanced the protection afforded by soluble antigen to adult mice as well as greatly increasing the T cell specific proliferative response, IFN-γ production and antibody levels. NISV are safe, stable, and inexpensive and promote TH1 and CD8$^+$ lymphocyte activation. In BALB/c dams vaccinated with NISV entrapped soluble antigen and infected on day 12 of pregnancy with 20 tissue cysts of *T. gondii* (RRA strain), congenital infection was reduced from a control level of 50% to 12% in surviving offspring and foetal death from 50% to nil. The identification of protective antigens in the soluble fraction is well advanced.

NATO ASI Series, Vol. H 78
Toxoplasmosis
Edited by Judith E. Smith
© Springer-Verlag Berlin Heidelberg 1993

Introduction

The recent demonstration that a live vaccine can successfully prevent parasite induced abortion in sheep [Buxton et al. 1991] has indicated the tremendous potential for successful vaccination against toxoplasmosis. However, a veterinary vaccine based on live organisms is undesirable and a safe non-living defined vaccine needs to be developed, most especially if it is to be used in humans. In recent years two parasite antigens have been identified as likely vaccine candidates, the major immunodominant membrane antigen P30 [Bulow and Boothroyd, 1991; Khan et al. 1991] and the excretory/secretory recombinant antigen P24 [Duquesne et al. 1991]. While vaccinating rats with P24 or with synthetic peptides derived from the primary structure of the molecule reduced mortality in animals infected with the virulent RH strain the ability of these vaccine candidates to reduce cyst burdens or prevent congenital toxoplasmosis awaits determination. P30, on the other hand, has been shown not only to protect against adult toxoplasmosis but also to exacerbate infection depending on which adjuvant is used [Kasper et al. 1985; Bulow and Boothroyd, 1991; Khan et al. 1991]. A further complication with P30 is that we have shown that a monoclonal antibody against P30, C1E3, which can passively transfer resistance to adults, can by itself induce abortion by mechanisms that are in the process of being identified [Alexander and Smith, in prep]. It is therefore imperative when developing a vaccine against toxoplasmosis to study the protection afforded both to the adult and the foetus in well characterised laboratory models of the disease.

In our laboratories we have recently demonstrated that the BALB/c mouse can be used as a model of human or ovine congenital *T. gondii* infection [Roberts and Alexander, 1992]. Infecting dams for the first time during the early period of gestation (day 7) results in foetal death, resorption or still birth. Although mortality falls if dams are infected later in pregnancy (day 12) at least 50% of all litter mates become infected. If however, BALB/c dams are infected several weeks before mating they develop immunity capable of protecting their embryos even if reinfection occurs during pregnancy. Ideally a successful vaccine should induce a similar level of protection. The induction of protective immunity is dependent on the nature of the immune response generated. Although antibodies have been shown to passively transfer protection [Johnson et al. 1983] the weight of evidence indicates that protective immunity against toxoplasmosis is mediated by CD8$^+$ lymphocytes [Gazzinelli et al. 1991, Parker et al. 1991, Khan et al. 1991]. However CD4$^+$ lymphocytes can influence infection [Parker et al. 1991; Vollmer et al. 1987] and protective immunity in vaccinated animals has been attributed to synergy between CD8$^+$ T cells and the Th1 CD4$^+$ subset [Gazzinelli et al. 1991]. Thus an adjuvant which promoted the activation of these T cell subsets would theoretically be an ideal component of a *T. gondii* subunit vaccine.

Using the laboratory disease models described above, and soluble antigen fractions entrapped in a non-ionic surfactant vesicles as a vaccine, we have successfully induced a high level of protection against adult acquired and congenital toxoplasmosis.

Materials and Methods

Mice   Inbred BALB/c and BALB/K mice and outbred Strathclyde A strain mice were maintained in this laboratory under conventional conditions. Mice were used when 8-10 weeks old and each experimental group comprised of 5-10 animals.

Infections   The brains of strain A mice, infected with the RRA (Beverley) strain of *T. gondii* 12 weeks previously, were used as a source of tissue cysts which were harvested and enumerated as previously described [Roberts and Alexander 1992]. All experimental infections were by the oral route and the congenital infection model was also as described previously [Roberts and Alexander 1992]. Briefly BALB/c mice were infected on days 11-12 of pregnancy with 20 tissue cysts. Surviving offspring were then transferred to infected foster mothers and the incidence of congenital infection measured 8-9 weeks after birth by ELISA. Severity of infection was monitored, where appropriate, by mortality levels or by total cyst counts in the brain.

Antigen Preparations   Freeze-thawed killed tachyzoites (kP), tachyzoite excretory/secretory antigens (ESAg), membrane antigens and soluble antigens (STAg) were all used in vaccination studies. *T. gondii* tachyzoites of the RH strain were obtained from peritoneal exudates of infected cotton rats and washed 3 times in saline. ESAg was obtained by incubating 5×10^{10} tachyzoites overnight in 40 mls of PBS. Tachyzoites were removed by centrifugation at

1000g and the supernatant collected. All protein concentrations were determined by a Bradford assay [Bradford 1976]. Tachyzoite soluble and membrane antigen fractions were obtained following disruption of $5x10^{10}$ parasites in hypotonic buffer (40ml 10mM Tris-HC1, 2mM EDTA, pH7.8) using a Brown homogeniser followed by centrifugation at 10,000G for 30 min at 4°C. The supernatant comprised the STAg and the pellet the membrane fraction. The membrane antigens were further purified using 1% octyl glucoside followed by centrifugation at 100,000G. The supernatant was collected and dialysed overnight against PBS at 4°C to remove the detergent.

Vaccine Preparations   All animals to receive vaccine preparations were inoculated subcutaneously with 50µg tachyzoite antigen 2 weeks and 4 weeks before infection. Antigen for vaccination was used either in a free form or emulsified in Freund's Complete Adjuvant or entrapped within a novel non-ionic surfactant vesicle formulation.

Vesicle Formation   Non-ionic surfactant vesicles (NSIV) were formed by the method of Brewer and Alexander [1992]. Briefly a mixture of the non-ionic surfactant 1-mono palmitoyl glycerol, Cholesterol Dicetyl phosphate [Sigma, Poole, Dorset, UK] were formed in PBS in the molar ratio 5:4:1 by the technique described by Collins et al. [1990]. Vesicle preparations were subsequently sonicated for 5 min at 20°C in a Mettler Electronics waterbath sonicator (50 Hz Pasadena, CA]. STAg entrapment into preformed vesicles was achieved by the dehydration-rehydration technique as described by Kirkby and Gregoriadis [1984]. Briefly, 5ml (150 µmol) of vesicle solution were mixed with 2ml STAg in PBS (5mg/ml) in polypropylene centrifuge tubes [Elkay Products Inc., Shrewsbury, MA] and flash frozen as a thin shell by swirling on liquid nitrogen. Preparations were then lyophilized in a freeze drier [Edwards high Vacuum, Crawley, Surrey, UK] at 0.1 torr overnight before rehydration in 0.5 ml distilled water. The samples were left to stand for 30 mins and then made up to 7 ml with distilled water. The vesicles were washed 3 times by centrifugation at 100,000g and the final entrapped protein concentration measured after vesicle lysis with propanol. The STAg concentration was adjusted to 500µg/ml for vaccination.

Results

In a series of experiments STAg was found consistently to provide significantly better ihibition of cyst growth than either whole killed tachyzoites or other tachyzoite antigen fractions. A representative experiment is shown [Fig. 1]. Preliminary experiments using STAg emulsified in FCA as a subcutaneous vaccine did not significantly reduce cyst burdens while two subcutaneous injections of FCA alone significantly increased cyst numbers in the brain (P<0.01) compared with control mice [Fig. 2].

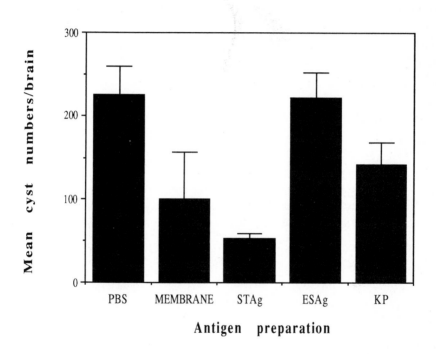

Fig 1   The mean number of cysts (+/- S.E.), 8 weeks post infection in the brains of BALB/c mice previously vaccinated subcutaneously with different antigen fractions (2x50μg) 2 weeks and 4 weeks before infection orally with 20 cysts.

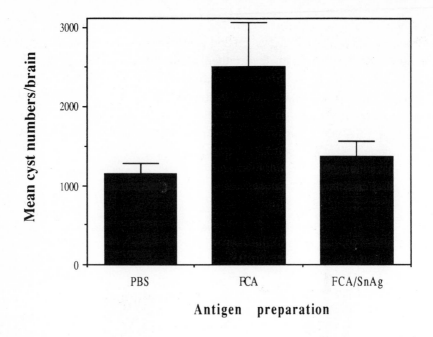

Fig2 The mean number of cysts (+/- S.E.), 6 weeks post infection, in the
brains of BALB/K mice infected orally with 20 cysts. Mice were
inoculated subcutaneously 2 weeks and 4 weeks before infection
with PBS, FCA or FCA containing 50µg STAg.

When the vaccine consisted of two subcutaneous inoculations of STAg
(P<0.05), STAg entrapped in NISV (P<0.01) or STAg mixed with NISV
(P<0.05) but not NISV alone cyst numbers were significantly reduced
compaed with control mice. However, STAg entrapped within NISV produced
significantly reduced cyst numbers compared with all other STAg vaccinated
groups [Fig. 3].
Vaccinating BALB/c mice with STAg entrapped in NISV 2 and 4 weeks before
mating resulted in greatly increased antibody levels [Fig. 4a] and significantly
reduced cyst numbers in the brains [Fig. 4b] some eight weeks after infection
compared with control animals. Mice were infected orally with 20 cysts on
day 11/12 of pregnancy as described. Of the pups born to STAg/NISV
vaccinated mice all survived and only 12% were infected while more than half

of the pups from non-vaccinated were dead at or within 24 hours of birth. Of the surviving offspring from this group more than 50% were also infected with *T. gondii* [Fig. 5].

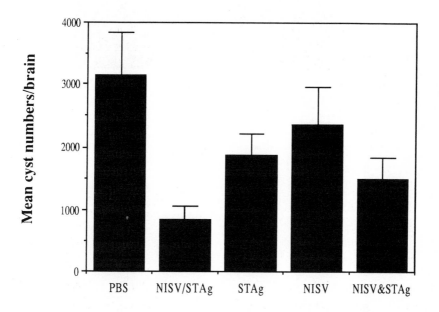

Fig3 The mean number of cysts (+/- S.E.), 4 weeks post infection in the brains of BALB/K mice infected orally with 20 cysts. Mice were inoculated subcutaneously 2 weeks and 4 weeks before infection with PBS, NISV entrapped STAg (NISV/STAg), STAg alone, NISV alone or NISV mixed with STAg (NISV&STAg).

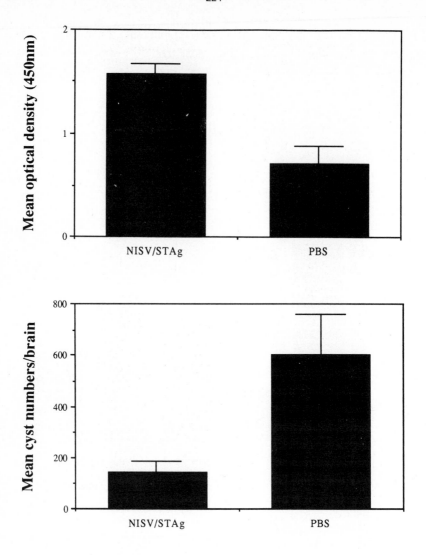

Fig4 The mean serum antibody levels (Fig4a) and mean cyst numbers
(+/- S.E.) in the brains (Fig4b) of BALB/c dams 8 weeks
post-infection with 20 cysts orally. The mice were infected on days
11-12 of pregnancy and the vaccinated group had been inoculated
with NISV/STAg (50μg) subcutaneously 2 weeks and 4 weeks
before infection.

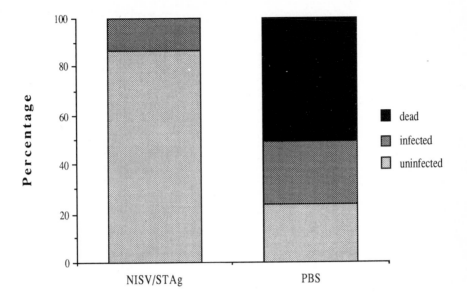

Fig5 The comparative fates of those offspring born to the BALB/c dams
described in Fig.4. The percentage of the surviving pups infected
with *T. gondii* was determined 8 weeks after birth by ELISA.

Discussion

Our results clearly demonstrate that the level of protective immunity induced
against *T. gondii* is not only associated wtih tachyzoite antigen subfraction
used but can be greatly enhanced or even inhibited by the adjuvant system
employed. FCA was found to inhibit the protective response induced by STAg
while protection was greatly enhanced using STAg entrapped in NISV. These
results parallel in many respects those reported earlier for the tachyzoite
membrane antigen P30 where FCA was found to exacerbate infections
following vaccination [Kasper et al. 1985] while the same antigen reconstituted
in liposomes, a vesicular system similar to NISV, promoted protection [Bulow
and Boothroyd, 1991].

Until recently the immunological mechanisms behind adjuvant activity were
poorly understood and certainly understudied. However, recent advances in

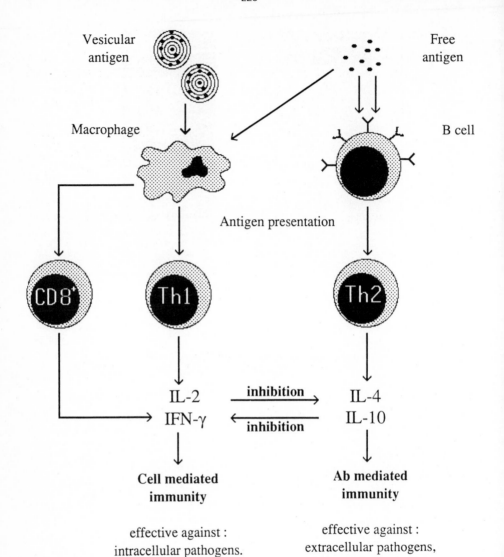

Fig6 Comparison of the proposed pathways of T cell activation using free soluble antigen or soluble antigen entrapped in non ionic surfactant vesicles.

our understanding of the cells and physiological signals, particularly cytokines [Coffman et al. 1991] involved in directing pathways of immunological activation have allowed greater insights as to how adjuvants may work. For example, as different antigen presenting cells (APC) provide the stimualtion and cofactors to promote different lymphocyte subsets [Bogan et al. 1991, Gajewski et al. 1991] it seems logical to assume that an adjuvant which stimulates or targets a particular APC could influence the direction of the immune response. Antigen presentation via macrophages has been associated with stimulation of the TH1 subset of $CD4^+$ lymphocytes rather than the TH2 subset which is optimally stimulated by B lymphocyes [Gajewski et al. 1991]. A vesicular adjuvant such as liposomes or NISV would undoubtedly favour a TH1 response as macrophages but not B cells internalise and process vesicular encapsulated antigen [Dal Monte and Szoka, 1989; Brewer and Alexander, 1992]. Macrophages, rather than B cells and dendritic cells, have also been shown to be the major cells for class I MHC restricted responses to foreign antigen [Debrick et al. 1991]. Even within a single APC population the nature of the adjuvant can dramatically influence the form of the immune response [Harding et al. 1991]. Thus acid resistant liposomes favour processing of antigens by macrophages for class II MHC presentation while acid sensitive liposomes allow processing for both class II and class I MHC presentation.

The NISV adjuvant formulation we have employed in this study targets macrophages and is acid sensitive. Consequently we have induced a strong Th1 and $CD8^+$ lymphocyte response against *T. gondii* which induces augmented levels of IFN-γ production *in vitro* [Roberts, Brewer and Alexander, in prep] and results in high levels of protection against *T. gondii in vivo*. The proposed mode of action of NISV in directing pathways of immunological activation against antigen is summarised diagrammatically in Fig. 6.

The effectiveness of our STAg vaccine formulation was particularly impressive when tested in the BALB/c congenital model. We have recently demonstrated that a previous infection with *T. gondii* prevents vertical disease transmission in this model even if the mice are infected for a second time during pregnancy [Roberts and Alexander, 1992]. While vaccination with NISV/STAg markedly reduces but does not give total protection against vertical disease transmission it does completely eliminate foetal death. We are currently identifying those antigens within the STAg fraction that are protective. Preliminary findings indicate a strong correlation between a 120kDa antigen and protection.

References

Bogen, S.A., Weinberg, D.S., Abbas, A.K. [1991] Histologic analysis of T lymphocyte activation in reactive lymph nodes. J Immunol 147: 1537-1541.

Brewer, J.M., Alexander, J [1992] The adjuvant activity of non-ionic surfactant vesicles (niosomes) on the BALB/c humoral response to bovine serum albumin. Immunol 75: 570-575.

Bradford, M.M. [1976] A rapid and sensitive method for the quantification of microgram quantities of protein utilizing the principle of protein-dye binding. Analyt Biochem 72: 248-254.

Bulow, R., Boothroyd, J.C. [1991] Protection of mice from foetal *Toxoplasma gondii* infection by immunisation with p30 antigen in liposomes. J Immunol 147: 3496-3500.

Buxton, D., Thomson, K., Maley, S., Wright, S., Bos, H.J. [1991] Vaccination of sheep with a live incomplete strain (S48) of *Toxoplasma gondii* and their immunity to challenge when pregnant. Veterinary Record 129: 89-93.

Coffman, R.L., Varkila, R., Scott, P., Chatelain, R. [1991] Role of cytokines in the differentiation of CD4$^+$ T-cell subsets in *in vivo*. Immunol Rev 123: 189.

Collins, M., Carter, K.C., Baillie, A.J. [1990] NISV formation of stibogluconate for canine leishmanisis. J. Pharm Pharmacol 42: P53.

Dal Monte, P., Szoka, F.C. [1989] Effect of liposome encapsulation on antigen presentation *in vivo* - comparison of presentation by macrophage and B cell tumours. J Immunol 142: 1437-1443.

Debrick, J.E., Campbell, P.A., Staerz, V.D. [1991] Macrophages as accessory cells for class I MHC restricted immune responses. J. Immunol 147: 2846-2851.

Duquesne, V., Aurvault, C., Gras-Masse, H., Boutillon, C., Darcy, F., Cesbron-Delauw, M.F., Tartar, A., Capron, A. [1991] Identification of T cell epitopes within a 23-kD antigen (P24) of *Toxoplasma gondii*. Clin exp Immunol 84: 527-534.

Gajewski, T.F., Pimnas, M., Wong, T., Fitch, F.W. [1991] Murine Th1 and Th2 clones proliferate optimally in response to distinct APC populations. J Immunol 146: 1750-1758.

Gazzinelli, R.T., Hakim, F.T., Heiny, S., Shearer, G.M., Sher A [1991] Synergistic role of CD4$^+$ and CD8$^+$ T lymphocytes in IFN-γ production and protective immunity induced by an attenuated *T. gondii* vaccine. J Immunol 146: 286-292.

Harding, C.V., Collins, D.S., Kanagwa, O., Unanue, E.R. [1991] Liposome encapsulated antigens engender lysosomal processing for Class II presentation and cytosolic processing for Class I presentation. J Immunol 147; 2860-2863.

Kasper, L.H., Currie, K.M., Bradley, M.S. [1985] An unexpected response to vaccination with a purified membrane tachyzoite antigen (p30) of *Toxoplasma gondii*. J Immunol 134: 3426-3431.

Khan, I.A., Ely, K., Kasper, L.H. [1991] A purified parasite antigen (p30) mediates CD8$^+$ T cell immunity against foetal *Toxoplasma gondii* infection in mice. J Immunol, 147: 3501-3506.

Kirby, C., Gregoriadia, G. [1984] Dehydration-rehydration vesicles: a simple method of high yield entrapment in liposomes. Biotechnology 2: 979-984.

Johnson, A.M. [1984] Strain-dependent, route of challenge-dependent murine susceptibility to toxoplasmosis. Z Parasitenkd 70: 303-309.

Parker, S.J., Roberts, C.W., Alexander, J [1991] CD8$^+$ T cells are the major lymphocyte subpopulation involved in the protective immune response to *Toxoplasma gondii* in mice. Clin exp Immunol 84: 207-212.

Roberts, C.W., Alexander, J [1992] Studies on a murine model of congenital toxoplasmosis: vertical disease transmission only occurs in BALB/c mice infected for the first time during pregnancy. Parasitol 04: 19-23.

Vollmer, T.L., Waldour, M.K., Steinman, L., Conley, F.K. [1987] Depletion of T-4$^+$ lymphocytes with monoclonal antibody reactivates toxoplasmosis in the central nervous system: a model of superinfection in AIDS. J Immunol 138: 3737.

DEVELOPMENT OF A LIVE VACCINE AGAINST OVINE TOXOPLASMOSIS

H.J.Bos
Intervet International by, Parasitology R & D
POB 31, 5830 Boxmeer, The Netherlands

A vaccine has been developed using strain S48, which has lost the ability both to form tissue cysts in intermediate hosts and oocysts in the cat. The tachyzoites, cultured *in vitro*, are injected intramuscularly into ewes at least 4 weeks prior to mating and provide good protection against abortion and barrenness. Safety and efficacy trials are discussed.

Ovine toxoplasmosis

Toxoplasmosis as a cause of perinatal mortality in sheep was first identified by Hartley et al. [1954, 1957] in New Zealand and is now recognized as an important cause of abortion and perinatal lamb losses in many parts of the world [Dubey & Towle, 1986]. Under field conditions susceptible (seronegative) sheep become infected following the ingestion of grass or hay contaminated with *Toxoplasma* oocysts from cat faeces [Blewett & Watson, 1983]. Infection of the ovine placenta and conceptus occurs when a non-immune sheep ingests oocysts while pregnant. Infection early in pregnancy is likely to cause fetal resorption and the ewes subsequently will be barren, whereas infection late in pregnancy (day 120 +) will usually result in the birth of a normal lamb which may be infected and become immune. Infection in midterm (days 50-120) will cause fetal death, mummification and abortion; the time from infection to abortion being about 40 days, similar to enzootic abortion (caused by *Chlamydia*). Characteristically, the placental cotyledons contained small white foci of necrosis. Microscopic lesions in the fetus develop in the brain, lung, liver, heart, kidney and spleen. They consist of small foci of necrosis surrounded by inflammatory cells and represent primary damage caused by the parasite but organisms are only rarely found. Specific antibody to *T. gondii* may be detected in the fetal circulation 30 days after initial infection of the ewe.

NATO ASI Series, Vol. H 78
Toxoplasmosis
Edited by Judith E. Smith
© Springer-Verlag Berlin Heidelberg 1993

Prevention and control

After infection with *T. gondii* cysts or oocysts most sheep are immune and will not abort during following pregnancies. Therefore controlled infection before mating (e.g. by exposure to a contaminated environment has been suggested (and practised) as a method to reduce losses. Another method studied at the Moredun Research Institute in Edinburgh [Buxton et al. 1988] is the prophylactic treatment of ewes during pregnancy by daily doses of 15 to 30 mg of monensin: an effective but expensive method.

Once an outbreak is observed in lambing sheep one can only dispose of dead lambs and infected placentas and disinfect pens if applicable. Cats should be kept away from cereals, hay and bedding that is to be used for pregnant sheep. Dubey [1981] showed that goats vaccinated with the non pathogenic coccidium *Hammondia hammondi* were protected against abortion and neonatal death induced by toxoplasmosis. Beverley et al. [1971] found partial protection against *toxoplasma*-induced abortion in sheep using a killed vaccine (RH strain lysate). Ewes were challenged subcutaneously with mouse brain cysts, an unusual route. Other experiments using inactivated vaccines in sheep have not been successful [e.g. Wilkins et al. 1978], although an experiment with iscoms showed some effect [Buxton et al. 1989].

In 1983 Wilkins & O'Connell described a vaccination trial in sheep using an "incomplete" strain (S48) which was not infective to cats and did not seem to form tissue cysts in intermediate hosts. When administered parenterally to breeding ewes 6 weeks before tupping it induced significant protection to *Toxoplasma* abortion. In experimental and field trials it has been shown that lambing percentages increased significantly and that there is an associated reduction in the number of "dry" ewes [O'Connell et al. 1988]. Further experiments to corroborate the data from New Zealand on safety and efficacy of strain S48 are described in this paper.

Strain S48

In 1958 the strain was isolated at Wallaceville Animal Research Centre, Upper Hutt, New Zealand, from foetal cotyledons of an aborted lamb and has since then been maintained by twice weekly intra-peritoneal passages in mice.

Since 1988/89 the vaccine ("Toxovax") has been produced and sold in New Zealand by MAFTech, Wallaceville. The strain has been deposited in the

ATCC under no.40447 and its use as a vaccine in sheep and goats has been patented (NZ patent no.220023, granted 10 May 1988).

S48 has an incomplete life cycle: during the many years of continuous mouse passages it has lost the ability to form tissue cysts or oocysts. This has been demonstrated in SPF lambs, in cats, and in mice (see safety experiments).

S48 is highly lethal for mice (and hamsters): doses higher than 10^4 are fatal within 5-6 days and even infection i.p. with a few tachyzoites does not cause chronic infection, but will eventually kill the mouse.

Production and quality control of the vaccine

The use of mouse passages for production holds the risk of viral contaminants, such as rodent viruses including retroviruses. Because of the short life of the vaccine full biosafety testing is not possible. Therefore, we had to adapt S48 to continuous *in vitro* cultivation and use a seed lot system. Continuous *in vitro* cultivation was achieved in Vero cell monolayers using roller bottles to produce at a large scale. Tachyzoites are harvested when a majority of the cells are infected or destroyed (> 50% CPE). The concentrated vaccine contains 10^8 tachyzoites in 5 ml solvens. Viability is determined using a vital stain (Trypan blue). Immediately before use the concentrated vaccine is diluted 20 x in a sucrose phosphate diluent. One dose of 2 ml contains 2 x 10^6 organisms and is injected intramuscularly or subcutaneously. Up to 95% loss of viable tachyzoites is allowed over a 3-week shelf life period, since 10^5 viable tachyzoites are known to provide optimal protection. Even 10^4 tachyzoites will still give satisfactory protection.

Master seed was produced, frozen down and stored in liquid nitrogen. Recovery is slow and after thawing master seed or preproduction seed it takes a few passages *in vitro* to be able to produce vaccine in sufficient quantities. The master seed has been shown to comply with the quality control requirements laid down in the bovine vaccine guidelines, concerning the absence of extraneous viruses and specific pathogens such as BVD, Aujeszky, Rabies, FMD, and *Brucella*. The final product testing includes: *Mycoplasma*, bacteria, fungi, extraneous viruses, BVD, safety in sheep, viability, potency in mice, and Vero cell penetration. A final or intermediate evaluation of tests is taken at 7 days to enable release after 1 week. In the next two weeks of shelf life at 4-6°C the number of viable tachyzoites in the vaccine normally drops to 20-30% of the initial number.

Freezing or freeze-drying of the vaccine has not yet been satisfactory for practical use.

Safety experiments
Of vital importance for registration of the product is the demonstration that S48 *per se* does not form tissue cysts in intermediate hosts, particularly in sheep. (It was already known that the mouse passaged vaccine does not prevent the formation of tissue cysts after infection with the wild type strains of *Toxoplasma*).
The following experiment was carried out in *Toxoplasma*-free reared SPF-lambs at the Moredun Institute (Edinburgh):
Group 1. 2 lambs were kept as non-infected controls:
Group 2. 10 lambs were infected s.c. with either 10^7 (5 x normal dose) Vero cell cultured S48 (V-vaccine) or a similar does of mouse passaged S48 (M-vaccine):
Group 3. 4 lambs were infected orally with 1000 oocysts of the virulent M3 strain:
The lambs were kept under SPF conditions and were monitored for febrile and serological responses. Six weeks p.i. the lambs were killed and screened for evidence of tissue cysts using three methods:
1. Direct microscopy of homogenized brain samples (Percoll concentration technique)
2. Pepsin digest of pooled diaphragms and psoas muscles were inoculated into mice and also the brain samples from method 1. The mice were killed 6 weeks after inoculation and tested for evidence of *Toxoplasma* infection, via microscopy of Percoll concentrated, homogenized mouse brains and anti-*T. gondii* IgG ELISA.
3. Thigh muscles and unused portions of lamb brain from each group were fed to SPF cats (2 cats per group; each cat consumed approx. 100g of muscle and 25g of brain).
The vaccinates (no difference was observed between the V and M vaccinates) showed an early febrile response as compared to the M3 group (Fig.1). This may be due not to the different strains but to the different stages used: tachyzoites and oocysts respectively. Antibody titres reached a plateau in the vaccinates already after 1 week and in the M3 group after 2 weeks (Fig.2).

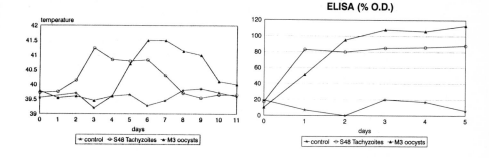

Fig 1. Safety trial. Febrile response after infection.

Fig 2. Safety trial. Antibody response after infection.

The results of examination of tissue samples are summarized in Table 1. All the mice inoculated with tissue from the non-infected and vaccinated lambs survived and remained seronegative, whereas all the mice inoculated with tissues from the M3 group became seropositive and died.

TABLE 1. Safety trial. Screening for tissue cysts.

	group 1 no infection	group 2 S48 infection	group 3 oocyst infection
microscopy: cysts in lamb brain	0/2*	0/10	2/4
infectivity of lamb tissue digest to mice: psoas diaphragm brain	0/10 0/10 -	0/20 0/18 0/20	- 2/2 6/6
serology in mice:	0/20	0/58	8/8

* No. positive/no. tested

The two cats fed tissue from the M3 infected lambs passed oocysts from day 5 until day 10. The other six cats (four in group 2 and two in group 1) remained negative.

Efficacy trials
Non-pregnant sheep model
Oral infection of sheep with *Toxoplasma* oocysts causes well-defined febrile and serological responses. Experiments at the Moredun Research Institute have shown that the febrile responses are consistently lower in medicated or immune sheep than in non-medicated or non-immune animals [Buxton et al. 1988; McColgan et al. 1988]. Febrile responses may therefore be used as an indicator of vaccine efficacy. It can be used as a preliminary screening and has the advantage of being based on the natural route of infection, not requiring pregnant ewes with longterm monitoring.

Using this model the effect of origin of the vaccine (mouse or *in vitro* culture) and age of the vaccine was tested. It appeared that vaccines of both origins were equally efficacious and that temperature responses after vaccination, but not the temperature responses after subsequent challenge, were dependent on age of the vaccine (i.e. number of viable tachyzoites; results not shown).

Challenge experiments in pregnant sheep
V and M vaccine
Scottish blackface and Swaledale ewes of various ages, and seronegative for *T. gondii* were vaccinated with 10^5 tachyzoites (2-week-old vaccine) produced either in mice (M-vaccine) or in Vero cells (V-vaccine). Oestrus cycles were synchronized and all animals were mated 77 days after vaccination. All the ewes were scanned by ultrasound 76 days after the first mating and the number of developing fetuses recorded. Groups were selected of the ewes that had held to the first service: 32 of each of the vaccinated groups (V and M), and 30 of the non-vaccinated. After 90 days of gestation all the animals were challenged orally with 2000 sporulated oocysts of the virulent M3 strain which represents a very heavy challenge infection. The groups were kept in 3 sheep houses, each containing 4 pens. Another group of 10 pregnant ewes was left unchallenged and the animals were distributed over the various pens (sentinel controls).

Both vaccines provided highly significant protection [Buxton et al. 1991]. Table 2 shows the lambing results. There was no significant difference between the M and V vaccinates with regard to the number of viable lambs born (av. lambing rate 76.6%), and mean gestation period was similar to that in the unchallenged controls.

TABLE 2. Challenge experiment. Lambing results.

Group	no. ewes	no. lambs expected	mean gestation	viable lambs (%)	nonviable lambs (%)
Toxovax M	32	47	144	34 (72.3)	13 (17.7)
Toxovax V	32	52	144	42 (80.8)	10 (19.2)
Challenge control	30	45	118*	8 (17.8)	37 (82.2)
Unchallenged	10	14	145	14 (100)	0 (0)

* significantly less than the other groups (P<0.001 by student's test)

In the non-vaccinated ewes, however, lambing rate was only 17.8% and the mean gestation period 118 days. A remarkable finding was that 65% of the precolostral lamb sera from the vaccinated ewes contained anti-*T. gondii* IgM antibodies and 53% specific IgG (Table 3). Lesions consistent with those seen in cases of *Toxoplasma* abortion were found in 46.8% of the placental cotyledons examined in the vaccinated groups. These observations are evidence of infection of the placenta and fetus with *T. gondii* in a large number of the vaccinated ewes, which is not associated with disease, mortality or abortion.

TABLE 3. Challenge experiment. Titres in precolostral lamb sera.

Group	no. tested	IgM positive (%)	IgM positive (%)
Toxovax V	40	27 (67.5)	21 (52.5)
Toxovax M	43	27 (62.8)	21 (52.5)
Challenge control	8	8 (100)	8 (100)
Unchallenged	14	0 (100)	0 (0)

Longterm efficacy of vaccine

A group of 27 ewes, vaccinated at the same time as described above, were challenged orally 18 months later with 2000 *T. gondii* (M3) oocysts when 89-91 days pregnant.

Antibodies to *T. gondii* peaked at 3-4 weeks, then decreased to a constant low level at 25 weeks after vaccination in this group (group 1) and rose rapidly after challenge (Fig. 3).

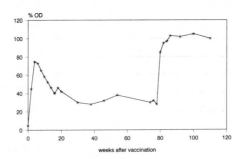

Fig 3. Longterm efficacy trial. Antibody responses during experiment.

Another group (group 2) of 34 non-vaccinated ewes were similarly challenged at the same stage of pregnancy while 12 control pregnant ewes (group 3) remained non-vaccinated and unchallenged.

Non-vaccinated ewes displayed a characteristic febrile response to challenge, whereas vaccinated animals showed a lower response, both earlier in onset and of shorter duration (Fig.4). Serologically group 2 showed a primary response to challenge infection which lagged two weeks behind the booster response seen in group 1 (Fig.5).

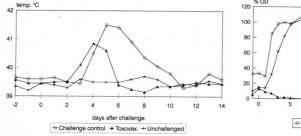

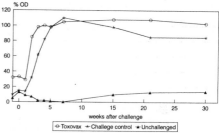

Fig 4. Longterm efficacy trial. Febrile responses after challenge.

Fig 5. Longterm efficacy trial. Antibody responses after challenge.

Again, lamb mortality in the vaccinated group was low (19.5%) compared with the non-vaccinated ewes in group 2 (88.9%). Serological and histopathological studies showed that all lambs in group 2 were born infected, compared with about half of those in group 1 and none in group 3.

Field Trials

A major field trial was carried out in the UK under the management of the Moredun Institute during the breeding season 1990/91 (under ATC 1708/0021). The vaccine was produced at Intervet UK in Cambridge at a dose rate of 10^6 viable tachyzoites per animal (Based on the assessment of stability experiments it was decided later to establish the dose rate at 2×10^6). Seventy five flocks were selected in Scotland, England and Wales, where at least 100 breeding replacments were being introduced per year, where *Toxoplasma* abortion had been diagnosed within the previous 3 years, and where seroprevalence for *T. gondii* among maiden ewes was $\leq 30\%$.

During phase 1 of the trial at least 100 maiden ewes were selected per flock, eartagged, blood-sampled and 50% vaccinated 4-6 weeks before tupping. Twenty percent of the blood samples were tested for IHA-titres to *T. gondii*.

During phase 2 the flocks were echo scanned 60-80 days after tupping and the number of foetuses recorded. Full abortion investigation took place and lambing records were kept. During phase 3 all 20 flocks in which *Toxoplasma* abortion occurred were bloodsampled again (all animals). Post-lambing samples paired with pre-mating samples provided data to assess the level of *Toxoplasma* challenge per flock.

Scanning records in the 20 flocks where *Toxoplasma* challenge occurred during pregnancy are shown in Table 4. There is a trend towards fewer barren ewes in the vaccinated group, but the difference is not significant.

TABLE 4. Field trial. Scanning records in 20 challenged flocks.

	vaccinated flocks	not vaccinated flocks
No. of barren ewes	58*	70*
Fetuses visible/100 ewes of the ram	157.85**	153.84**
no. of ewes scanned	1154	1130

* and **: differences not statistically significant.

TABLE 5. Field trial. Lambing results in 73 flocks. No. of lambs per 100
ewes put to the ram.

	vaccinated flocks	non vaccinated flocks
not challenged (n=48)	129.36	128.24
challenged by Toxoplasma (n=25)**	147.34*	137.01*

*   difference statisitcally significant (P<0.0001)
**   including 5 flocks in which multiple causes of abortion were diagnosed.

Lambing results in 73 (of the 75 selected) flocks are shown in Table 5. The
vaccinated group within the challenged flocks had significantly higher lambing
percentages than the non-vaccinated group. Remarkable is the fact that the
flocks challenged with *Toxoplasma* had significantly higher lambing
percentages than the unchallenged flocks. Due to between-farm variation
(accounting for 75-90% of all variance), arising from breed variety, type of
management and nutrition, it is not possible to regard the challenged or the
unchallenged population as a whole.
The level of challenge was generally low. In the 20 flocks where challenge
occurred only 10-14% of the ewes appeared to be challenged (i.e.
seronconversion from IHA-titre <1/160 to >1/640).   In one flock an
"abortion storm" was observed, with 13.6% *Toxoplasma* (or *Toxoplasma*
suspect) abortions in the non-vaccinated ewes and 3% in the vaccinated ewes.
All together in this trial involving over 11,000 maiden ewes of which 50%
were vaccinated, challenge with *Toxoplasma* during pregnancy occurred in
20% of the flocks. In these flocks 90% of the ewes showed no evidence of
being challenged, 72 cases of *Toxoplasma* abortion were diagnosed in the
non-vaccinated ewes and 29 cases in the vaccinated ewes: a significant
reduction in the vaccinated group (P<0.005, Fischers Exact test). There was
no evidence that vaccination influenced production in non-challenged flocks.
The non-vaccinated ewes that were seronegative post-lambing (approx. 70%)
are still susceptible to *Toxoplasma* abortion in the next breeding season,
whereas the vaccinated ewes will most likely be protected (see the chapter on
long term efficacy of the vaccine).

Discussion

Long-lived immunity to toxoplasmosis is presumably associated with persistent ('chronic') infection, i.e. the presence of tissue cysts, containing large numbers of bradyzoites. Immunity, humoral and cellular, is directed against the tachyzoite stage, that infects and destroys large numbers of cells in various tissues and organs. Bradyzoites, on the other hand, escape from attack by immune cells and, thus, represent a well-adapted mode of survival of the parasite.

Strains that do not form tissue cysts (bradyzoites), such as S48 and others like the temperature sensitive stain ts-4 [Pfefferkorn & Pfefferkorn, 1976], do not persist in the body of the host and, yet, cause long-lived immunity, in the absence of challenge infection.

Infection is usually aquired by the oral route (uptake of tissue cysts in meat or of oocysts in contaminated feed). Immunity indiced by S48, which is administered parenterally, is systemic and will not stop the initial development of intestinal (subclinical) stages. When the tachyzoites spread into the body by the blood stream to the liver, lungs, heart, and brain, and via lymphatics to regional lymph nodes and other organs and start to multiply, they will be attacked by antibodies and immune cells. During acute infection in pregnant females, the placenta and fetus will be infected. In vaccinated individuals the number of tachyzoites reaching the placenta and causing transplacental infection will be reduced substantially and will subsequently transform to bradyzoites (tissue cysts) which escape from immune attack. This hypothetical course of events may explain the observations in our challenge experiments.

If S48 tachyzoites completely disappear from the vaccinated animals, as is also suggested by recent PCR studies at the Moredun Institute, memory cells must remain present. As T-cell immunity seems to be of key importance [Krahenbuhl & Remington, 1982] the search for pretective T-cell stimulating antigens or epitopes is essential for future research towards a subunit or vector vaccine, particularly for use in humans.

Meanwhile a live attenuated vaccine, such as Toxovax, is a valuable tool in reducing the economic damage in sheep and goats, caused by toxoplasmosis. It fulfills most of the criteria put forward for a successful vaccine, such as low biohazard (safety for the operator and the consumer), absence of adverse effects in the host, duration of immunity, ease of large-scale production, and low production costs, and is, therefore, contradictory with earlier expressed expectations [Johnson, 1989]. Stability is still a major, albeit more logistic problem, but this may be resolved.

Acknowledgements
The author wishes to thank Dr. T. Schetters for critically reading the text and Ms Helma van Daal for preparing the print-ready manuscript.

References
Beverley J.K.A., Archer J.F., Watson W.A., Fawcett A.R., (1971) Trial of a killed vaccine in the prevention of ovine abortion due to toxoplasmosis. Brit Vet J 127: 529-535.
Blewett D.A., Watson W.A., (1983) The epidemiology of ovine toxoplasmosis. II Possible sources of infection in outbreaks of clinical disease. Brit Vet J 139: 546-555.
Buxton D., Blewett D.A., Trees A.J., McColgan C., Finlayson J. (1988) Further studies in the use of monensin in the control of experimental ovine toxoplasmosis. J Comp Path 88: 225-236.
Buxton D., Uggla A., Lovgren K., Thomson K., Lunden A., Morein B., Blewett D.A., (1989) Trial of a novel experimental Toxoplasma iscom vaccine in pregnant sheet. Brit Vet J 145: 451-457.
Buxton D., Thomson K., Maley S., Wright S., Bos H.J., (1991) Vaccination of sheep with a live incomplete strain (S48) of *Toxoplasma gondii* and their immunity to challenge when pregnant. The Vet Rec 129: 89-93.
Dubey J.P., (1981) Prevention of abortion and neonatal death due to toxoplasmosis by vaccination of goats with the nonpathogenic coccidium *Hammondia hammondi*. Am J Vet Res 42: 2155.
Dubey J.P., Towle A. (1986) Toxoplasmosis in sheep: A review and annotated bibliography. Misc Publ No 10, Commonwealth Institute of Parasitology, London 1986.
Hartley W.J., Jebson J.L., McFarlane D. (1954) New Zealand type II abortion in ewes. Austr Vet J 30: 216-218.
Hartley W.J., Marshall S.C. (1957) Toxoplasmosis as a cause of ovine perinatal mortality. N Z Vet J 5: 119-124.

Johnson A.M., (1989) Toxoplasma vaccines. In: Veterinary
protozoan and hemoparasite vaccines (ed Wright I G). CRC Press Inc,
Boca Raton, Florid: 177-203.

Krahenbuhl J.L., Remington J.S., (1982) The immunology of
Toxoplasma and toxoplasmosis. In: Immunology of parasitic
infections, 2nd ed (Cohen S, Warren K S eds), Blackwell Scientific,
Oxford.

McColgan C., Buxton D., Blewett, D.A. [1988] Titration of *Toxoplasma
gondii* oocysts in non-pregnant sheep and the subsequent challenge
during pregnancy. The Vet Rec 123: 467-470.

O'Connell E., Wilkins M.F., Te Punga W.A., (1988) Toxoplasmosis in
sheep. II. The ability of a live vaccine to prevent lamb losses after an
intravenous challenge with Toxoplasma gondii. N Z Vet J 36: 1-4.

Pfefferkorn E R, Pfefferkorn L C (1976) *Toxoplasma gondii*: isolation and
preliminary characterization of temperature-sensitive mutants. Exp Parasit
39: 365-376.

Wilkins M.F., O'Connell E. (1983) Effect of lambing percentage of
vaccinating ewes with *Toxoplasma gondii*. N Z Vet J 31: 181-182.

GENETIC REGULATION OF *TOXOPLASMA GONDII* INFECTION: INFLUENCE OF *LSH/ITY/BCG* GENE.

Jenefer M. Blackwell[1], Craig W. Roberts[2], Tamara I.A. Roach[1], James Alexander[2].

[1]   Department of Medicine, Level 5, Addenbrooke's Hospital, Hills Road, Cambridge CB2 2QQ, U.K.

[2]   Department of Immunology, University of Strathclyde, The Todd Centre, 31 Taylor Street, Glasgow G4 0NR, U.K.

The murine chromosome 1 gene *Lsh/Ity/Bcg* gene was identified nearly 20 years ago for its role in controlling the early phase of infection with *Salmonella typhimurium* and *Leishmania donovani*, and later as a major regulator of mycobacterial infections including *Mycobacterium bovis* BCG. Functional macrophage studies have shown that *Lsh* regulates macrophage priming activation for antimicrobial activity via the TNF-α dependent production of reactive nitrogen intermediates. Differential regulation of TNF-α is observed in bone marrow-derived macrophages from *Lsh* congenic mouse strains in response to both lipopolysaccharide and mycobacterial lipoarabinomannan, and when macrophages are plated onto the extracellular matrix proteins fibronectin and fibrinogen. The former accounts for the induction *Lsh* resistance mechanism by the infecting microorganism. The latter explains differential *Lsh* gene expression in macrophages in different tissue sites *in vivo*, in particular in the viscera versus the skin. Since macrophages are an important host cell in *Toxoplasma gondii* infection, and *T. gondii* is known to elicit a strong TNF-α response, we thought it would be of interest to examine this infection in *Lsh* congenic mouse strains.

Following oral administration of 20 brain cysts of the RRA strain, mice carrying the *Lsh* resistant allele on a B10 genetic background showed significantly higher mortality over the acute (first 10 days) phase of infection than B10 *Lsh* susceptible mice. Although mortality in both strains was accompanied by an increase in serum TNF-α levels, administration of neutralising rabbit anti-TNF-α did not significantly enhance survival suggesting that other inflammatory mediators were responsible for the acute mortality observed. *Lsh* resistant mice which survived the acute phase of infection went on to have significantly lower brain cyst loads than B10 *Lsh* susceptible mice. Infection intraperitoneally (i.p.) led to delayed mortality, with the mean time to 50% mortality being significantly longer in *Lsh* resistant than *Lsh* susceptible mice. On a BALB genetic background, it was the i.p. route of infection which led to acute mortality and more rapid death in the *Lsh* resistant strain. Interestingly, when the i.p. parasite inoculum was reduced and mortality delayed, *Lsh* susceptible mice died more rapidly and i.p. administration of rabbit anti-TNF-α led to 100% mortality between days 8 and 10 of infection in both strains, consistent with a critical protective role for TNF-α during this phase of infection. Overall these results show that the *Lsh* gene may play different modulating roles over the course of *T. gondii* infection depending on the potency of the inoculum and the route and kinetics of infection.

ESTABLISHING A LABORATORY FOR PARASITE GENOME ANALYSIS: FOCUS ON THE PARASITIC PROTOZOA *TOXOPLASMA*, *TRYPANOSOMA* AND *LEISHMANIA*.

Jenefer M. Blackwell, James W. Ajioka and Sara E. Melville

University of Cambridge, Department of Pathology, Tennis Court Road, Cambridge CB2 1PQ.

Over the past twelve months we have been working towards the establishment of a new laboratory for Parasite Genome Analysis at the University of Cambridge, U.K. This laboratory will build on, and provide new tools for, research addressing specific biological problems, but taking on board the philosophy of other major (e.g. human, *Drosophila, Caenorhabditis elegans*) genome projects which provide a major resource for the international research community. The major aims of the initiative are:-
1. To establish a laboratory for Parasite Genome Analysis in Cambridge concentrating initially on production of Yeast Artifical Chromosome (YAC) and dual purpose shuttle vector/mapping pacmid P1 and cosmid libraries for the protozoan parasites *Toxoplasma, Trypanosoma*, and *Leishmania*. High density filters will be produced for mapping purposes and made available to the international research community. A central mapping database will be established in Cambridge.

2. To develop a series of PCR-based sequence tagged site (STS), polymorphic STS (pSTS), expression tagged site (ETS) markers to provide genetic and physical mapping tools which can be used to analyse genetic/phenotypic/karyotypic variation in natural populations of these parasites.

3. To use, and make generally available, the mapping and dual purpose shuttle vector/mapping libraries as a major resource in addressing specific biological problems by reverse genetics.

4. To exploit these parasite genomes, where the chromosomes are resolvable by pulse-field gel electrophoresis and the genome sizes are two orders of magnitude smaller then mammalian genomes, as models to address broader questions relating to the evolution and organization of eukaryote genomes.

MUCOSAL IMMUNE RESPONSE IN TOXOPLASMOSIS

D. Bout, T. Chardès, M.N. Mévelec, D. Buzoni-Gatel, F. Velge-Roussel, I. Dimier, I. Bourguin, N. Debard,
Unite de Recherche Université-INRA d'Immunologie Parasitaire et CJF INSERM, UFR des Sciences Pharmaceutiques de Tours et Station de Pathologie Infectieuse et Immunologie, Centre INRA de Tours, F-37380 Nouzilly.

Infection with *T. gondii* most commonly occurs via the oral route. Ingested organisms are released from cysts or oocysts within the gastrointestinal tract, invade the intestinal epithelium and are disseminated throughout the body. The local immune system is now accepted as acting as a protective barrier against various infectious agents and strategies for developing efficient oral vaccines are currently being investigated. In order to design such a vaccine through a rational approach, a better knowledge of the mucosal acquired immune response, initiation and effectors, is a prerequisite.

We first monitored the kinetics of the IgA antibody response in serum, intestinal secretions and milk from orally infected mice. About 60% of the intestinal anti *T. gondii* IgA response involved secretory IgA. These IgA antibodies mostly recognized three antigens (SAG1, GRA4, ROP2) which could be good candidates for vaccination.

Peyer patches and mesenteric lymphocyte blastogenic response to a toxoplasma sonicate occured on day 6 and then rapidly decreased. Splenic blastogenic stimulation began during week 4 and persisted throughout the experiment (13 weeks). The mesenteric response was dominated by a Th2-type cytokine pattern whereas a predominant Th1 cytokine response was observed in the spleen.

We also demonstrated that 1) rat small intestine epithelial cell line IEC-6 could be activated by IFN gamma to inhibit the intracellular replication of *T. gondii*, and 2) oral infection of CBA mice stimulated parasite-specific cytotoxic intraepithelial lymphocytes. This could be of relevance as a first line defence against *Toxoplasma* infection.

Finally, the adjuvant effect of cholera toxin on the mucosal immune response was tested for protection. Oral immunization with *T. gondii* antigens in association with cholera toxin induced enhanced protective, humoral and cell-mediated immunity in sensitive C57BL/6 mice.

References

1) T. Chardès et al., Infect. Immun. [1990] 58, 1240-1246.
2) I. Bourguin et al., FEMS Microbiol Lett. [1991] 81, 265-272.
3) M.N. Mévèlec et al., Mol. Biochem. Parasitol. [1992] 56, 227-238.
4) T. Chardès et al., Immunology [1992] 78, 421-429.
5) I. Dimier, D. Bout, Eur. J. Immunol. [1993] 23, 981-983.
6) I. Bourguin et al. Infect. Immun. [1993] 61, 2082-2088.

ANTENATAL SCREENING FOR TOXOPLASMOSIS IN TURKIYE

Ugur Dilmen[1] MD; I. Safa Kaya[1], MD; Ugur Ciftci[2], Ph.D; Eflatun Goksin[3], MD.

Turkish Health and Therapy Foundation, Department of Neonatology[1], Microbiology[2], and Obstetrics and Gynecology[3], Ankara, Turkiye.

A total of 1772 pregnant women were screened during the first eight weeks of pregnancy by the toxoplasma hemogglutination (HA) test. The frequency of infection as determined by the toxoplasma HA test is seen in Table 1.

TABLE 1. The prevelance of toxoplasma HA test.

Titer	Number	%
Negative (<1/16)	620	34.9
1/16	122	6.8
1/32	212	11.9
1/64	190	10.7
1/128	189	10.6
1/256	234	13.2
>1/512	205	11.5

Using this assay we found that 66% of all cases examined had positive antibody titres. The remainder were followed by the toxoplasma HA test once a month during pregnancy prospectively. 7 individuals seroconverted (1%), during weeks 12, 17, 20, 24, 28 and 32 of gestation. *Toxoplasma* IgM ELISA tests also proved positive in these cases. Spiramycin was administered to seroconverted cases. Toxoplasma IgM in the cord blood was negative in all cases. Antenatal ultrasonographic follow up and postnatal physical examination were within normal limits.

TOXOPLASMOSIS IN GREECE: SEROLOGICAL STUDIES

S. Kanelli-Papaioannou, Institut Pasteur Hellenique, Department of Parasitology, 127, Vas Sofias Ave, GR 11521, Athens, Greece.

Over the last three years, 6,707 sera have been examined for antibodies against *Toxoplasma gondii*. These samples were taken from individuals all over Greece.

The human sera came from patients both with and without the classical features associated with toxoplasma infection such as fever, eye damage, lymph node infection, and immunodepression. Patients ranged from new born babies up to 75 years old.

Serological methods used were the Dye-Test and indirect immunofluorescence for the determination of total antibodies and the TOXO-ISAGA for the determination of IgM antibodies.

Results: From the 6,707 sera examined, 2800 (41.74%) were found to have antibodies against toxoplasmosis.

IgM antibodies were found in 472 (10.05%) sera via the TOXO-ISAGA method, from patients with recent toxoplasmosis infection.

Due to the high sensitivity of the above method, IgM antibodies were found in some patients after a 2-3 year period. To overcome this problem, a second sample is taken and analysed after a 3 week period.

Future work includes diagnosis of congenital toxoplasmosis with IgA antibody detection and also the detection of the parasite with the use of Polymerase Chain Reaction (PCR).

CRITICAL EVALUATION OF IGA ANTIBODIES AS AN INDICATION OF EARLY TOXOPLASMA-INFECTION.

Hanns M. Seitz, Inst. of Medical Parasitology, University of Bonn, Germany.

The risk of a toxoplasma infected pregnant woman having a baby infected with *toxoplasma* is virtually zero, if the mother was infected before conception. If the woman has her first test for toxoplasma specific antibodies during pregnancy it may be difficult to judge the time of infection and the possible risk for fetal damage.

Many cases can be clarified by determination of IgM antibodies but in a fraction of the mothers the IgM persists for a year, or even longer, making interpretation difficult.   Recently tests for IgA were introduced into the diagnosis of toxoplasmosis. It was said, that high IgA titers are found in the early stages of the infection only.

We tested sera from 409 individuals using an IgA capture test based on the principle of the ISAGA-tests. For comparison we performed the IgM-ISAGA, the IgM-LIFT and the dye test.

One observation was that there was absolute agreement on all negative sera and in the sera with low titers.

For some sera we had information on the appearance of lymphadenopathy in the donor as an indication of a very recent infection. Two individuals for example showed high titers (1:4000 and 1:16000) eleven and fourteen weeks after the observation of lymph-adenopathy, as expected they were negative three months later. Contrary to this finding other patients presented "irregular" results:

a. low or negative titers early in infection (three weeks to two months after lymphadenopathy) while having high IgM titers at the same time or

b. in two other individuals moderate to high IgA titers persisting for six months or more with IgM tests being negative.

These results indicate that the determination of the IgA antibodies is not the ultimate solution in *toxoplasma* diagnosis because - as with other tests - deviations from the normal pattern occur making the interpretation of the titer values difficult.

EXPRESSION OF *TOXOPLASMA GONDII* GENES IN rBCG

Louis M. Weiss M.D., M.P.H.[1,2] Herbert B. Tanowitz M.D.[1,2], Murray Wittner Ph.D.[2], William Jacobs Jr. Ph.D.[3,4]
[1] - Division of Infectious Diseases, Department of Medicine
[2] - Division of Parasitology, Department of Pathology
[3] - Department of Microbiology and Immunology
[4] - Howard Hughes Medical Institute

Albert Einstein College of Medicine
1300 Morris Park Avenue
Bronx, New York, 10461, U.S.A.

Toxoplasma gondii (Tg) is a well described ubiquitous intracellular Apicomplexan protozoan parasite of mammals and birds responsible for several clinical diseases in man, including congenital infection in normal hosts and encephalitis in patients with AIDS. Cell mediated immunity is now felt to be of primary importance for providing protection from Tg infection. In order to generate cell mediated immune responses to cloned Tg antigens we have expressed Tg cDNA clones in BCG vectors. Live recombinant BCG (rBCG) cells expressing foreign antigen genes have been shown to generate both humoral and cellular immune responses (both helper and cytotoxic) to the expressed genes. Initially a Tg cDNA clone reactive to a Tg specific Mab 92-10b was isolated from a gt11 library and subcloned into pMV261.

Sequence analysis has shown this cDNA Tg clone is GRA-1 (p24). pMV261 is a mycobacterial shuttle vector with a kanamycin resistance selectable marker, the *E. coli* plasmid replicon derived from pUC19 (oriE), a mycobacterial plasmid replication segment (oriM) as well as an expression cassette containing a mycobacterial promoter (HSP), multiple cloning site and transcription terminator. This vector expresses inserted genes as a fusion protein with HSP and is expressed in both *E. coli* and BCG. The fusion protein is found in the cytoplasm of BCG when expressed. A rBCG clone expressing the Mab92-10b antigen (GRA-1) was obtained and used to immunize CD-1 mice. Partial protection with an increased time to death on challenge with 10,000 RH strain tachyzoites was seen in rBCG:Tg immunized mice compared to mice immunized with BCG alone. We have used rPCR to clone from mRNA the genes for SAG-1 (p30) and SAG-2 (p22) and are using the same technique for GRA-2 (p28.5) and ROP-2. Expression in BCG using pMV2619S seq to allow expression of the recombinant genes on the surface of BCG is also in progress. Such rBCG:Tg constructs may be useful in vaccination (oral, subcutaneous or intravenous) as well as in studies of antigen processing of isolated Tg genes *in vitro*.

INDEX

Printing: Druckhaus Beltz, Hemsbach
Binding: Buchbinderei Schäffer, Grünstadt

NATO ASI Series H

NATO ASI Series H

NATO ASI Series H

NATO ASI Series H

NATO ASI Series H